2. Greek yogurt with berries

Ingredients:

- 1 cup plain Greek yogurt (low•fat or non•fat)
- 1/2 cup mixed berries (such as blueberries, raspberries, blackberries)
- 1 tsp honey (optional)

Instructions:

1. Spoon the Greek yogurt into a bowl or serving dish.

2. Top the yogurt with the mixed berries.

3. If desired, drizzle the honey over the top.

That's it! This makes a quick, easy, and nutritious snack or light meal.

Some benefits of this recipe:

- Greek yogurt is high in protein, which can help keep you feeling full.
- Berries are packed with antioxidants, fiber, and other beneficial nutrients.
- The honey adds a touch of sweetness if desired, but is optional.

This is a great option for someone who has had gastric bypass surgery, as it's gentle on the stomach, nutrient•dense, and easy to digest. Adjust the portion sizes as needed to meet your individual dietary needs and preferences.

3. Cottage cheese with pineapple

Ingredients:

- 1 cup low•fat or non•fat cottage cheese
- 1/2 cup diced fresh pineapple
- 1 tsp honey (optional)

Instructions:

1. Scoop the cottage cheese into a bowl or serving dish.

2. Top the cottage cheese with the diced pineapple.

3. If desired, drizzle the honey over the top.

That's all there is to it! This makes a quick, easy, and healthy snack or light meal.

Some benefits of this recipe:

- Cottage cheese is high in protein, which can help keep you feeling full.
- Pineapple is a good source of vitamin C, fiber, and bromelain (an enzyme that may aid digestion).
- The honey adds a touch of sweetness if desired, but is optional.

This is a great option for someone who has had gastric bypass surgery, as it's gentle on the stomach, nutrient•dense, and easy to digest. The cottage cheese and pineapple combination provides a nice balance of protein, carbohydrates, and fiber. Adjust the portion sizes as needed to meet your individual dietary needs and preferences.

Welcome to the ***"High-Protein Gastric Bypass Cookbook: 110+ Tasty and Nutritious Recipes"!*** This book is designed to be your comprehensive guide to enjoying delicious, high-protein meals that support your nutritional needs following gastric bypass surgery.

Undergoing gastric bypass surgery is a life-changing decision that sets you on a path toward improved health and well-being. However, the journey doesn't end with the surgery itself. Adjusting to a new lifestyle and diet is crucial for long-term success. Proper nutrition plays a vital role in ensuring your body receives the essential nutrients it needs while promoting healing and aiding in weight management.

In this cookbook, we've curated over 110 recipes that are not only high in protein but also full of flavor and variety. These recipes are tailored to meet the unique dietary requirements of gastric bypass patients, focusing on easy digestion, balanced nutrition, and enjoyable eating experiences. From hearty breakfasts and satisfying lunches to delectable dinners and delightful snacks, each recipe is crafted to help you thrive on your post-surgery journey.

Why High-Protein?

After gastric bypass surgery, your stomach's capacity is significantly reduced, and your body's ability to absorb nutrients changes. Protein becomes a cornerstone of your diet, aiding in muscle maintenance, tissue repair, and overall health. High-protein meals help you feel fuller for longer, support your metabolic rate, and contribute to maintaining lean body mass as you lose weight.

Each recipe includes detailed nutritional information, serving sizes, and easy-to-follow instructions to make your cooking experience as seamless as possible. We've also included tips and modifications to cater to different stages of your post-surgery diet, ensuring you have options no matter where you are on your journey.

A Healthier Future Awaits

Embarking on a post-gastric bypass lifestyle can be challenging, but with the right tools and support, it's entirely achievable. This cookbook aims to be a valuable resource in your kitchen, inspiring you to create meals that nourish your body and delight your taste buds. Whether you're a seasoned cook or new to the culinary world, these recipes are designed to be accessible, enjoyable, and, most importantly, beneficial to your health.

*Thank you for choosing the **"High-Protein Gastric Bypass Cookbook: 110+ Tasty and Nutritious Recipes."** Here's to a healthier, happier you! Enjoy your culinary adventure and the delicious path to wellness.*

1. Scrambled eggs with spinach

Ingredients:

- 3 large eggs
- 1/4 cup egg whites
- 1 cup fresh spinach, chopped
- 1 tbsp low•fat milk or unsweetened almond milk
- 1 tbsp grated parmesan cheese
- Salt and pepper to taste

Instructions:

1. In a small bowl, whisk together the whole eggs, egg whites, and milk until well combined.

2. Heat a non•stick skillet over medium heat and spray with a small amount of cooking spray.

3. Add the chopped spinach and sauté for 1•2 minutes until wilted.

4. Pour the egg mixture into the skillet and let sit for 20•30 seconds to set the bottom.

5. Using a spatula, gently push the eggs from the side of the pan into the center, tilting the pan to allow the uncooked egg to flow to the edges.

6. Continue this process until the eggs are mostly set but still look a bit moist.

7. Remove from heat and stir in the parmesan cheese. Season with salt and pepper to taste.

8. Serve immediately. This recipe makes 1 serving.

The combination of whole eggs, egg whites, and spinach provides a high protein, nutrient•dense meal that is gentle on the stomach after gastric bypass surgery. Adjust portions as needed to meet your individual dietary needs.

4. Protein pancakes with almond flour

Ingredients:

- 1/2 cup almond flour
- 2 large eggs
- 1/4 cup unsweetened almond milk
- 1 scoop (about 30g) vanilla protein powder
- 1 tsp baking powder
- 1/4 tsp cinnamon (optional)
- Butter or non•stick cooking spray for cooking

Instructions:

1. In a medium bowl, whisk together the almond flour, eggs, almond milk, protein powder, baking powder, and cinnamon (if using) until a smooth batter forms.

2. Heat a non•stick skillet or griddle over medium heat and grease with a small amount of butter or cooking spray.

3. Scoop the batter onto the hot surface, using about 2•3 tablespoons per pancake.

4. Cook for 2•3 minutes per side, or until the pancakes are golden brown and cooked through.

5. Serve the protein pancakes warm, with your choice of toppings such as fresh berries, a drizzle of sugar•free syrup, or a spoonful of Greek yogurt.

This recipe makes approximately 4•5 small pancakes.

The almond flour and protein powder provide a boost of protein to help keep you feeling full, while the eggs and almond milk keep the pancakes moist and tender. This is a great option for those following a high•protein diet after gastric bypass surgery. Adjust the portion size as needed to meet your individual dietary requirements.

5. Smoothie with protein powder, spinach, and berries

Ingredients:

- 1 cup unsweetened almond milk
- 1 scoop (about 30g) vanilla or unflavored protein powder
- 1 cup fresh spinach leaves
- 1/2 cup frozen mixed berries (such as blueberries, raspberries, blackberries)
- 1 tbsp ground flaxseed (optional)
- Ice cubes (optional)

Instructions:

1. Add the almond milk, protein powder, spinach, frozen berries, and flaxseed (if using) to a high•powered blender.

2. Blend on high speed until the mixture is smooth and creamy, about 1•2 minutes.

3. If a thicker consistency is desired, add a few ice cubes and blend again briefly.

4. Pour the smoothie into a glass and enjoy immediately.

This smoothie provides a nutritious and filling meal or snack, with a balance of protein, fiber, and healthy fats. The spinach and berries add important vitamins, minerals, and antioxidants.

The protein powder helps to keep you feeling full and satisfied, which is important for those who have had gastric bypass surgery. Adjust the amount of protein powder used based on your individual protein needs.

You can also experiment with different types of protein powder, such as whey, casein, or plant•based varieties, to find the one that works best for you. Enjoy this smoothie as a quick and easy way to get a nutrient•dense boost!

6. Egg white omelette with vegetables

Ingredients:

- 1/2 cup egg whites (about 4•5 large egg whites)
- 1/4 cup diced bell pepper
- 1/4 cup diced onion
- 1/2 cup spinach or kale, chopped
- 1 tbsp grated low•fat cheddar cheese (optional)
- Salt and pepper to taste
- Cooking spray

Instructions:

1. Crack the egg whites into a small bowl and whisk lightly with a fork until frothy.

2. Spray a non•stick skillet with cooking spray and heat over medium heat.

3. Add the diced bell pepper and onion to the skillet and sauté for 2•3 minutes until softened.

4. Pour the egg whites into the skillet and let them sit for 20•30 seconds to set the bottom.

5. Using a spatula, gently push the cooked egg from the sides into the center, tilting the pan to allow the uncooked egg to flow to the edges.

6. Continue this process until the eggs are mostly set but still look a bit moist.

7. Add the chopped spinach or kale to one half of the omelet and fold the other half over on top.

8. Sprinkle the grated cheese over the top, if using.

9. Cook for an additional 1•2 minutes until the cheese is melted and the omelet is cooked through.

10. Slide the omelet onto a plate and season with salt and pepper to taste.

This high•protein, veggie•packed omelet is a great option for those following a gastric bypass diet. The egg whites provide a lean source of protein, while the vegetables add important nutrients and fiber. Adjust the portion size as needed to meet your individual dietary needs.

7. Quinoa breakfast bowl with nuts and seeds

Ingredients:

- 1/2 cup cooked quinoa, cooled
- 1/4 cup unsweetened almond milk
- 1 tbsp chopped walnuts
- 1 tbsp chopped almonds
- 1 tbsp pumpkin seeds
- 1 tbsp chia seeds
- 1 tsp honey (optional)
- Cinnamon to taste

Instructions:

1. In a medium bowl, combine the cooked quinoa and almond milk. Stir to combine.

2. Top the quinoa mixture with the chopped walnuts, almonds, pumpkin seeds, and chia seeds.

3. If desired, drizzle the honey over the top and sprinkle with cinnamon.

That's it! This makes a delicious and satisfying breakfast bowl.

The benefits of this recipe include:

- Quinoa is a high•protein, gluten•free grain that provides complex carbohydrates and fiber.
- Nuts and seeds offer healthy fats, protein, and additional fiber.
- The almond milk and optional honey provide creaminess and a touch of sweetness.
- Cinnamon is a warming spice that may help regulate blood sugar levels.

This breakfast bowl is gentle on the stomach, nutrient•dense, and easy to digest • making it an excellent choice for someone following a gastric bypass diet. Adjust the portion sizes as needed to meet your individual dietary requirements.

8. Chia pudding with protein powder

Ingredients:

- 1/4 cup chia seeds
- 1 cup unsweetened almond milk
- 1 scoop (about 30g) vanilla or unflavored protein powder
- 1 tsp honey (optional)
- 1/2 tsp vanilla extract
- Pinch of cinnamon (optional)

Instructions:

1. In a medium bowl, whisk together the chia seeds, almond milk, protein powder, honey (if using), vanilla extract, and cinnamon (if using) until well combined.

2. Cover the bowl and refrigerate for at least 2 hours, or overnight, stirring occasionally, until the mixture has thickened to a pudding•like consistency.

3. Divide the chia pudding into individual serving bowls or containers.

4. Top with your choice of fresh berries, chopped nuts, or a drizzle of nut butter, if desired.

This chia pudding is a great option for a high•protein, nutrient•dense breakfast or snack after gastric bypass surgery. The chia seeds provide fiber, protein, and healthy omega•3 fatty acids, while the protein powder helps to keep you feeling full and satisfied.

The almond milk and optional honey add creaminess and a touch of sweetness. Feel free to experiment with different protein powder flavors or mix•in toppings to find your favorite combination.

Adjust the portion size as needed to meet your individual dietary requirements. This recipe makes approximately 2 servings.

9. Tofu scramble with vegetables

Ingredients:

- 1 block (14 oz) firm or extra•firm tofu, drained and crumbled
- 1 tbsp olive oil
- 1/2 cup diced bell pepper
- 1/2 cup diced onion
- 1 cup chopped spinach or kale
- 2 tbsp nutritional yeast
- 1 tsp garlic powder
- 1 tsp ground cumin
- 1/4 tsp turmeric (optional, for color)
- Salt and pepper to taste

Instructions:

1. Heat the olive oil in a large non•stick skillet over medium heat.

2. Add the diced bell pepper and onion to the skillet and sauté for 3•4 minutes until softened.

3. Crumble the tofu into the skillet and use a spatula to break it up into small pieces.

4. Stir in the nutritional yeast, garlic powder, cumin, and turmeric (if using). Season with salt and pepper to taste.

5. Continue cooking, stirring occasionally, for 5•7 minutes until the tofu is heated through and the vegetables are tender.

6. Add the chopped spinach or kale to the skillet and cook for an additional 2•3 minutes, until the greens are wilted.

7. Serve the tofu scramble warm, on its own or with a side of roasted potatoes or whole grain toast.

This tofu scramble is a great high•protein, vegetarian option for those following a gastric bypass diet. The tofu provides a good source of plant•based protein, while the vegetables add important nutrients and fiber. Adjust the portion size as needed to meet your individual dietary requirements.

10. Oatmeal with protein powder and nuts

Ingredients:

- 1/2 cup old•fashioned rolled oats
- 1 cup unsweetened almond milk
- 1 scoop (about 30g) vanilla or unflavored protein powder
- 1 tbsp chopped walnuts
- 1 tbsp chopped almonds
- 1 tsp honey (optional)
- Cinnamon to taste

Instructions:

1. In a small saucepan, combine the rolled oats and almond milk. Bring to a simmer over medium heat, stirring occasionally.

2. Once the oats have softened and the mixture has thickened, 5•7 minutes, remove from heat.

3. Stir in the protein powder until fully incorporated and the oatmeal is smooth and creamy.

4. Top the oatmeal with the chopped walnuts and almonds.

5. If desired, drizzle the honey over the top and sprinkle with cinnamon.

This high•protein oatmeal makes a satisfying and nutritious breakfast. The combination of oats, protein powder, and nuts provides a balance of complex carbohydrates, protein, and healthy fats to help keep you feeling full and satisfied.

The benefits of this recipe include:

- Oats are a good source of fiber, which can be beneficial for those with a gastric bypass.
- Protein powder helps to increase the protein content of the meal.
- Nuts add healthy fats, fiber, and additional protein.
- The optional honey provides a touch of sweetness.

Adjust the portion size and amount of protein powder as needed to meet your individual dietary requirements. This recipe makes 1 serving.

11. Hard•boiled eggs

Ingredients:

• 6 large eggs

Instructions:

1. Place the eggs in a single layer in a saucepan and cover with cold water by 1 inch.

2. Bring the water to a boil over high heat. Once the water reaches a full boil, remove the pan from the heat and cover.

3. Let the eggs sit in the hot water for the following times:
   • For soft•boiled eggs: 6•7 minutes
   • For hard•boiled eggs: 12 minutes

4. Drain the hot water and cover the eggs with cold water to stop the cooking process.

5. Let the eggs sit in the cold water for 5 minutes.

6. Peel the eggs and enjoy as is, or use them in other recipes.

Hard•boiled eggs are an excellent high•protein, nutrient•dense option for those following a gastric bypass diet. They are easy to digest, portable, and can be prepared in advance for quick snacks or meals.

Some benefits of hard•boiled eggs include:

• High in protein, which can help keep you feeling full and satisfied.
• Contain important vitamins and minerals like vitamin A, vitamin B12, and selenium.
• The yolks provide healthy fats and choline, which is important for brain health.

Adjust the portion size as needed to meet your individual dietary requirements. Hard•boiled eggs can be stored in the refrigerator for up to 1 week.

12. Edamame

Ingredients:

- 1 lb frozen edamame in the pod
- 1 tsp coarse sea salt (or to taste)

Instructions:

1. Bring a large pot of water to a boil over high heat.

2. Add the frozen edamame pods to the boiling water and cook for 5•7 minutes, until the pods are bright green and tender.

3. Drain the edamame and transfer to a serving bowl.

4. Sprinkle the coarse sea salt over the edamame and toss to coat.

5. Serve the edamame warm, providing a small bowl for discarding the empty pods.

That's it! This simple preparation allows the natural flavors of the edamame to shine.

Edamame is an excellent high•protein, nutrient•dense snack option for those following a gastric bypass diet. Some key benefits include:

- High in protein, with about 17 grams per 1 cup serving
- Good source of fiber, vitamins, and minerals
- Low in calories and carbohydrates
- Gentle on the stomach and easy to digest

Adjust the portion size as needed to meet your individual dietary requirements. Edamame can be enjoyed on its own as a snack or incorporated into other dishes.

Remember to discard the empty pods after eating the edamame beans inside. Enjoy this simple, healthy snack!

13. Hummus with cucumber slices

Ingredients:

- 1 (15 oz) can chickpeas, drained and rinsed
- 2 tbsp tahini
- 2 tbsp fresh lemon juice
- 1 garlic clove, minced
- 2 tbsp olive oil
- 1/4 tsp ground cumin
- Salt and pepper to taste
- 1 medium cucumber, sliced into rounds

Instructions:

1. In a food processor or high•powered blender, combine the drained chickpeas, tahini, lemon juice, garlic, olive oil, and cumin. Blend until smooth and creamy.

2. Season the hummus with salt and pepper to taste.

3. Arrange the cucumber slices on a serving plate or platter.

4. Scoop the hummus into a bowl and serve alongside the cucumber slices for dipping.

This hummus is a great high•protein, nutrient•dense option for those following a gastric bypass diet. The chickpeas provide a good source of plant•based protein, while the tahini, olive oil, and lemon juice add healthy fats and flavor.

The fresh cucumber slices provide a refreshing, low•calorie vehicle for enjoying the hummus. The combination of protein, fiber, and hydration from the cucumber can help promote feelings of fullness.

Adjust the portion sizes as needed to meet your individual dietary requirements. This recipe makes approximately 1 cup of hummus, which can be served with the cucumber slices as a snack or light meal.

14. Protein bars (low sugar)

Ingredients:

- 1 cup rolled oats
- 1/2 cup unsweetened shredded coconut
- 1/2 cup vanilla protein powder
- 1/4 cup natural peanut butter (or other nut butter)
- 1/4 cup unsweetened applesauce
- 2 tbsp honey
- 1 tsp vanilla extract
- 1/4 tsp salt

Instructions:

1. Line an 8x8 inch baking pan with parchment paper and set aside.

2. In a large bowl, mix together the rolled oats, shredded coconut, and protein powder.

3. In a separate bowl, combine the peanut butter, applesauce, honey, vanilla extract, and salt. Stir until well blended.

4. Pour the wet ingredients into the dry ingredients and mix until a thick, sticky dough forms.

5. Press the dough evenly into the prepared baking pan.

6. Refrigerate for at least 2 hours, or until firm.

7. Remove the bars from the pan by lifting the parchment paper. Cut into 8 equal bars.

These low•sugar protein bars are a great option for those following a gastric bypass diet. They provide a balance of protein, complex carbs, and healthy fats to help keep you feeling full and satisfied.

The benefits include:

- High in protein from the protein powder and nut butter
- Low in added sugars, using honey as the main sweetener
- Fiber from the oats and coconut
- Portable and easy to grab as a snack

Store the protein bars in an airtight container in the refrigerator for up to 1 week. Adjust the portion size as needed to meet your individual dietary requirements.

15. Cottage cheese with sliced peaches

Ingredients:

- 1 cup low•fat or non•fat cottage cheese
- 1 medium peach, sliced

Instructions:

1. Scoop the cottage cheese into a bowl or serving dish.

2. Arrange the sliced peach on top of the cottage cheese.

That's it! This simple combination makes a delicious and satisfying snack or light meal.

The benefits of this recipe include:

- Cottage cheese is high in protein, which can help keep you feeling full and satisfied.
- Peaches are a good source of fiber, vitamins, and antioxidants.
- The combination of protein and fruit provides a balanced and nutrient•dense option.
- Cottage cheese and peaches are gentle on the stomach, making this a great choice for those following a gastric bypass diet.

Adjust the portion sizes as needed to meet your individual dietary requirements. This recipe makes 1 serving.

You can also try this with other types of fresh fruit, such as berries, nectarines, or plums, depending on your preferences and what is in season.

16. Turkey roll•ups with avocado

Ingredients:

- 4 oz sliced turkey breast
- 1/2 medium avocado, sliced
- 1 tbsp plain Greek yogurt
- 1 tsp Dijon mustard
- Salt and pepper to taste

Instructions:

1. In a small bowl, mix together the Greek yogurt and Dijon mustard until well combined.

2. Lay the turkey slices out flat on a clean surface. Spread a thin layer of the yogurt•mustard mixture over each slice.

3. Place a few slices of avocado near the edge of each turkey slice.

4. Carefully roll up the turkey slices around the avocado, securing them with toothpicks if needed.

5. Arrange the turkey roll•ups on a plate and season with salt and pepper to taste.

That's it! This makes a simple, yet satisfying high•protein snack or light meal.

The benefits of this recipe include:

- Turkey is a lean source of protein, which is important for those following a gastric bypass diet.
- Avocado provides healthy fats, fiber, and nutrients like potassium.
- The Greek yogurt and Dijon mustard add creaminess and flavor without a lot of extra calories or sugar.
- The compact roll•up format makes this a convenient and easy•to•eat option.

Adjust the portion sizes as needed to meet your individual dietary requirements. This recipe makes 4 turkey roll•ups.

17. Greek yogurt with a handful of nuts

Ingredients:

- 1 cup plain Greek yogurt (high in protein)
- 1 handful of mixed nuts (such as almonds, walnuts, pecans)

Instructions:

1. Scoop the Greek yogurt into a bowl.

2. Top the yogurt with a handful of mixed nuts.

Nutrition Information:

- Calories: Approximately 250•300 calories (depending on the type and amount of nuts used)

- Protein: Around 20•25 grams of protein from the Greek yogurt

- Healthy Fats: The nuts provide heart•healthy unsaturated fats

- Fiber: The nuts add some fiber to the dish

This simple Greek yogurt and nut combination is an excellent high•protein, nutrient•dense snack or light meal for someone following a gastric bypass diet. The protein and healthy fats from the Greek yogurt and nuts can help promote feelings of fullness and satiety.

Some tips:
- Choose plain, unsweetened Greek yogurt to minimize added sugars.
- Go for a variety of nuts like almonds, walnuts, pecans, or pistachios to get a mix of nutrients.
- Start with a small portion of nuts, as they are calorie•dense.
- This can be enjoyed on its own or paired with other high•protein foods.

Let me know if you need any other gastric bypass friendly recipe ideas!

18. Protein shake with almond milk

Ingredients:

- 1 cup unsweetened almond milk
- 1 scoop (about 30g) vanilla or unflavored protein powder
- 1/2 cup frozen berries (such as blueberries, raspberries, or strawberries)
- 1 tbsp almond butter (or peanut butter)
- 1 tsp honey (optional)
- Ice cubes (optional)

Instructions:

1. Add the almond milk, protein powder, frozen berries, almond butter, and honey (if using) to a high•powered blender.

2. Blend on high speed until the mixture is smooth and creamy, about 1•2 minutes.

3. If a thicker consistency is desired, add a few ice cubes and blend again briefly.

4. Pour the protein shake into a glass and enjoy immediately.

This protein shake provides a nutrient•dense and filling option for those following a gastric bypass diet. The benefits include:

- High in protein from the protein powder to help keep you feeling full.
- Almond milk is low in calories and carbs, yet provides healthy fats and calcium.
- Frozen berries add natural sweetness, fiber, and antioxidants.
- Almond butter provides additional protein and healthy fats.
- The optional honey adds a touch of sweetness if desired.

Adjust the amount of protein powder and other ingredients based on your individual dietary needs and preferences. This recipe makes one serving.

Enjoy this protein shake as a quick and easy meal or snack option after gastric bypass surgery.

19. Macaroni and Cheese

Ingredients:

- 8 oz elbow macaroni
- 3 tbsp butter
- 3 tbsp all•purpose flour
- 2 cups milk
- 2 cups shredded cheddar cheese
- 1/2 tsp salt
- 1/4 tsp black pepper

Instructions:

1. Bring a large pot of salted water to a boil. Cook the macaroni according to package instructions until al dente. Drain and set aside.

2. In a medium saucepan, melt the butter over medium heat. Whisk in the flour and cook for 1•2 minutes, stirring constantly, to make a roux.

3. Gradually whisk in the milk. Bring the mixture to a simmer and cook, stirring frequently, until thickened, about 5 minutes.

4. Remove the sauce from heat and stir in 1 1/2 cups of the shredded cheddar cheese until melted and smooth. Season with salt and pepper.

5. Add the cooked macaroni to the cheese sauce and stir to combine.

6. Transfer the macaroni and cheese to a baking dish. Top with the remaining 1/2 cup shredded cheddar cheese.

7. Bake at 375°F for 15•20 minutes, until the cheese on top is melted and bubbly.

8. Let stand for 5 minutes before serving.

Enjoy your homemade, creamy macaroni and cheese! You can customize it by adding extras like bacon, broccoli, or breadcrumbs on top.

20. Tuna salad on cucumber slices

Ingredients:

- 1 (5 oz) can of water•packed tuna, drained
- 2 tbsp plain Greek yogurt
- 1 tbsp diced celery
- 1 tbsp diced red onion
- 1 tsp Dijon mustard
- 1 tsp lemon juice
- Salt and pepper to taste
- 1 medium cucumber, sliced into rounds

Instructions:

1. In a small bowl, combine the drained tuna, Greek yogurt, celery, red onion, Dijon mustard, and lemon juice. Mix well until fully incorporated.

2. Season the tuna salad with salt and pepper to taste.

3. Arrange the cucumber slices on a serving plate or platter.

4. Scoop a small amount of the tuna salad onto each cucumber slice, spreading it evenly.

That's it! This makes a simple, yet nutritious and satisfying snack or light meal.

The benefits of this recipe include:

- Tuna is an excellent source of lean protein, which is important for those following a gastric bypass diet.
- Greek yogurt adds creaminess and extra protein to the tuna salad.
- Cucumber slices provide a refreshing, low•calorie base that is gentle on the stomach.
- The combination of protein, fiber, and hydration from the cucumber can help promote feelings of fullness.

Adjust the portion sizes as needed to meet your individual dietary requirements. This recipe makes approximately 8•10 tuna salad•topped cucumber slices.

21. Grilled chicken breast with steamed broccoli

Ingredients:

- 4 oz boneless, skinless chicken breast
- 1 tsp olive oil
- Salt and pepper to taste
- 1 cup broccoli florets
- 1 tbsp lemon juice (optional)

Instructions:

1. Preheat your grill or grill pan to medium•high heat.

2. Brush the chicken breast with the olive oil and season with salt and pepper.

3. Grill the chicken for 4•6 minutes per side, or until it reaches an internal temperature of 165°F.

4. While the chicken is grilling, steam the broccoli florets in a steamer basket or a small saucepan with a bit of water for 5•7 minutes, until tender•crisp.

5. Remove the chicken from the grill and let it rest for a few minutes.

6. Serve the grilled chicken breast alongside the steamed broccoli. Drizzle the broccoli with a squeeze of lemon juice, if desired.

This grilled chicken and steamed broccoli dish is an excellent option for a gastric bypass diet. It's high in protein, low in carbs, and provides a good source of fiber and essential vitamins and minerals from the broccoli.

Some tips:
- Choose boneless, skinless chicken breasts to keep the fat and calorie content low.
- Adjust the portion size of chicken to your individual needs, as 4•6 oz is a typical serving.
- Steam the broccoli instead of sautéing or roasting it to keep the preparation simple and low•calorie.
- Experiment with different seasoning blends or lemon juice to add flavor without adding extra calories.
- Serve this dish with a small portion of a low•carb vegetable side, such as roasted cauliflower or a side salad.

This grilled chicken and steamed broccoli is a quick, easy, and nutritious meal option for a gastric bypass diet. It's a great way to incorporate lean protein and fiber•rich vegetables into your daily routine.

22. Turkey and cheese roll•ups

Ingredients:

- 4 oz thinly sliced turkey breast
- 2 oz low•fat cheddar or Swiss cheese, sliced
- 1 tbsp Dijon mustard
- 1 tbsp chopped fresh parsley (optional)

Instructions:

1. Lay the turkey slices out flat on a clean surface.

2. Place a slice of cheese on each turkey slice.

3. Spread a thin layer of Dijon mustard over the cheese.

4. Carefully roll up the turkey slices, enclosing the cheese inside.

5. Secure the roll•ups with toothpicks or cut them into bite•sized pieces.

6. Sprinkle the roll•ups with chopped parsley, if desired.

Nutrition Information (per serving, 2 roll•ups):
- Calories: 150•180
- Protein: 20•25g
- Fat: 6•8g
- Carbs: 2•3g
- Fiber: 0•1g

These turkey and cheese roll•ups are an excellent option for a gastric bypass diet. They are high in protein, low in carbs, and provide a satisfying snack or light meal. The combination of lean turkey and cheese makes them a great source of nutrients.

Some tips:
- Choose thinly sliced, low•sodium turkey breast to keep the sodium content low.
- Opt for low•fat or reduced•fat cheese to keep the fat and calories in check.
- Adjust the portion size to your individual needs, as 2•3 roll•ups can make a satisfying snack.
- Serve the roll•ups with a side of non•starchy vegetables, such as cucumber or bell pepper slices, for added nutrients.

These turkey and cheese roll•ups are easy to prepare, portable, and can be enjoyed as a quick and nutritious option on a gastric bypass diet.

23. Lentil soup

Ingredients:

- 1 tbsp olive oil
- 1 onion, diced
- 2 carrots, peeled and diced
- 2 celery stalks, diced
- 3 garlic cloves, minced
- 1 cup dried brown or green lentils, rinsed
- 4 cups low•sodium chicken or vegetable broth
- 1 (14.5 oz) can diced tomatoes
- 1 tsp dried thyme
- 1 tsp dried oregano
- Salt and pepper to taste
- Chopped fresh parsley for garnish (optional)

Instructions:

1. In a large pot or Dutch oven, heat the olive oil over medium heat. Add the onion, carrots, and celery. Sauté for 5•7 minutes, until the vegetables are softened.

2. Add the garlic and sauté for an additional minute, until fragrant.

3. Stir in the lentils, broth, diced tomatoes, thyme, and oregano. Season with salt and pepper to taste.

4. Bring the soup to a boil, then reduce the heat and let it simmer for 20•25 minutes, or until the lentils are tender. Ladle the soup into bowls and garnish with chopped fresh parsley, if desired.

This lentil soup is an excellent option for a gastric bypass diet. It's high in protein and fiber, low in fat, and packed with nutrient•dense vegetables. The combination of lentils, broth, and spices makes it a satisfying and comforting meal.

Some tips:
- Use low•sodium broth to keep the sodium content in check.
- Adjust the portion size to your individual needs, as a 1•cup serving can be a satisfying meal.
- Serve the soup with a side salad or roasted non•starchy vegetables for added nutrients.
- This soup can be made in advance and stored in the refrigerator or freezer for easy meal prep.

Lentil soup is a great option for a gastric bypass diet, providing a balance of protein, fiber, and complex carbohydrates to help keep you feeling full and satisfied.

24. Salmon salad with mixed greens

Ingredients:

- 4 oz cooked salmon fillet, flaked
- 2 cups mixed greens (such as spinach, arugula, kale)
- 1/4 cup cherry tomatoes, halved
- 2 tbsp sliced cucumber
- 1 tbsp diced red onion
- 1 tbsp olive oil
- 1 tbsp lemon juice
- Salt and pepper to taste

Instructions:

1. In a large salad bowl, combine the flaked salmon, mixed greens, cherry tomatoes, cucumber, and red onion.

2. In a small bowl, whisk together the olive oil and lemon juice. Season with a pinch of salt and pepper.

3. Drizzle the dressing over the salad and gently toss to coat.

Nutrition Information (per serving):
- Calories: 200•250
- Protein: 20•25g
- Fat: 12•15g
- Carbs: 5•10g
- Fiber: 3•5g

This salmon salad is an excellent option for a gastric bypass diet. It's high in protein from the salmon, low in carbs, and packed with nutrient•dense greens and vegetables. The healthy fats from the salmon and olive oil help promote feelings of fullness.

Some tips:
- Choose wild•caught salmon for more omega•3 fatty acids.
- Adjust the portion size of salmon to your individual needs.
- Add extra non•starchy veggies as desired.
- Use a light vinaigrette or lemon juice•based dressing to keep it low•calorie.

This salmon salad can be enjoyed as a main dish or a side salad. It's a great way to incorporate lean protein, healthy fats, and fiber•rich greens into your gastric bypass diet.

25. Chicken and vegetable stir•fry

Ingredients:

- 1 lb boneless, skinless chicken breasts, cut into 1•inch pieces
- 2 tbsp low•sodium soy sauce
- 1 tsp sesame oil
- 1 tbsp olive oil
- 2 cloves garlic, minced
- 1 inch piece fresh ginger, grated
- 2 cups mixed vegetables (such as broccoli, bell peppers, snap peas, mushrooms)
- 1/4 cup low•sodium chicken broth
- 1 tsp cornstarch
- Salt and pepper to taste
- Chopped green onions for garnish (optional)

Instructions:

1. In a bowl, combine the chicken, soy sauce, and sesame oil. Toss to coat and let marinate for 15•20 minutes.

2. Heat the olive oil in a large skillet or wok over high heat.

3. Add the garlic and ginger and stir•fry for 30 seconds, until fragrant.

4. Add the marinated chicken and stir•fry for 3•4 minutes, until the chicken is lightly browned.

5. Add the mixed vegetables and stir•fry for an additional 3•4 minutes, until the vegetables are tender•crisp.

6. In a small bowl, whisk together the chicken broth and cornstarch. Pour the mixture into the skillet and stir to coat the chicken and vegetables.

7. Cook for 1•2 minutes, until the sauce has thickened slightly.

8. Season with salt and pepper to taste. Serve the chicken and vegetable stir•fry immediately, garnished with chopped green onions if desired.

This chicken and vegetable stir•fry is an excellent option for a gastric bypass diet. It's high in protein from the chicken, low in carbs, and packed with fiber•rich vegetables. The combination of lean protein, non•starchy vegetables, and a light sauce makes it a satisfying and nutrient•dense meal.

26. Turkey chili

Ingredients:

- 1 lb ground turkey
- 1 onion, diced
- 3 cloves garlic, minced
- 1 bell pepper, diced
- 2 cans (15 oz each) black beans, rinsed and drained
- 1 can (15 oz) diced tomatoes
- 1 can (6 oz) tomato paste
- 2 cups low•sodium chicken or vegetable broth
- 2 tsp chili powder
- 1 tsp ground cumin
- 1 tsp dried oregano
- 1/2 tsp smoked paprika
- Salt and pepper to taste
- Chopped fresh cilantro for garnish (optional)

Instructions:

1. In a large pot or Dutch oven, cook the ground turkey over medium•high heat, breaking it up with a wooden spoon, until browned and cooked through, about 5•7 minutes.

2. Add the diced onion, garlic, and bell pepper to the pot. Sauté for 3•4 minutes, until the vegetables are softened.

3. Stir in the black beans, diced tomatoes, tomato paste, broth, chili powder, cumin, oregano, and smoked paprika. Season with salt and pepper to taste.

4. Bring the chili to a simmer and let it cook for 20•25 minutes, stirring occasionally, until the flavors have melded and the chili has thickened. Ladle the turkey chili into bowls and garnish with chopped fresh cilantro, if desired.

This turkey chili is an excellent option for a gastric bypass diet. It's high in protein from the ground turkey, packed with fiber•rich beans and vegetables, and low in fat. The combination of lean protein, complex carbohydrates, and spices makes it a satisfying and nutrient•dense meal.

Some tips:
- Use low•sodium broth and canned beans to keep the sodium content in check.
- Adjust the portion size to your individual needs, as a 1•cup serving can be a satisfying meal.
- Serve the chili with a side of non•starchy vegetables, such as a small salad or roasted cauliflower, for added nutrients.
- This chili can be made in advance and stored in the refrigerator or freezer for easy meal prep.

27. Quinoa and black bean salad

Ingredients:

- 1 cup cooked quinoa, cooled
- 1 (15 oz) can black beans, rinsed and drained
- 1 cup diced cucumber
- 1/2 cup diced red bell pepper
- 1/4 cup diced red onion
- 2 tbsp chopped fresh cilantro
- 2 tbsp lime juice
- 1 tbsp olive oil
- 1/2 tsp ground cumin
- Salt and pepper to taste

Instructions:

1. In a large bowl, combine the cooked quinoa, black beans, cucumber, bell pepper, red onion, and cilantro.

2. In a small bowl, whisk together the lime juice, olive oil, and cumin. Season with a pinch of salt and pepper.

3. Pour the dressing over the quinoa and bean mixture and toss gently to coat.

4. Refrigerate for at least 30 minutes to allow the flavors to meld.

5. Serve chilled or at room temperature.

This quinoa and black bean salad is an excellent option for a gastric bypass diet. It's high in protein and fiber, low in fat, and packed with nutrient•dense ingredients. The combination of quinoa, black beans, and vegetables provides a satisfying and filling meal.

Some tips:
- Use pre•cooked or instant quinoa to save time.
- Adjust the portion size to your individual needs.
- Add extra vegetables, such as diced tomatoes or avocado, for additional nutrients.
- This salad can be enjoyed on its own or served over a bed of mixed greens.

This quinoa and black bean salad is a great make•ahead option for a gastric bypass diet. It's easy to prepare, nutritious, and can be enjoyed as a main dish or a side.

28. Egg salad lettuce wraps

Ingredients:

- 6 hard•boiled eggs, peeled and chopped
- 2 tbsp plain Greek yogurt
- 1 tbsp Dijon mustard
- 1 tbsp chopped fresh dill (or 1 tsp dried dill)
- 1 tbsp finely chopped red onion
- Salt and pepper to taste
- 4•6 large lettuce leaves (such as romaine or butter lettuce)

Instructions:

1. In a medium bowl, combine the chopped hard•boiled eggs, Greek yogurt, Dijon mustard, dill, and red onion. Mix well until fully incorporated.

2. Season the egg salad with salt and pepper to taste.

3. Lay the lettuce leaves flat on a clean surface. Scoop a portion of the egg salad onto the center of each lettuce leaf.

4. Carefully wrap the lettuce around the egg salad, creating a lettuce wrap.

5. Serve the egg salad lettuce wraps immediately.

These egg salad lettuce wraps are an excellent option for a gastric bypass diet. They are high in protein from the eggs, low in carbs, and provide a satisfying and nutrient•dense snack or light meal.

Some tips:
- Use plain, unsweetened Greek yogurt to keep the calorie and sugar content low.
- Adjust the portion size of egg salad to your individual needs, as 2•3 lettuce wraps can make a satisfying snack.
- Choose large, sturdy lettuce leaves, such as romaine or butter lettuce, to easily wrap the egg salad.
- Add extra vegetables, such as diced cucumber or tomato, for additional nutrients.
- Serve the egg salad lettuce wraps with a side of non•starchy vegetables, such as carrot or celery sticks, for a more complete meal.

These egg salad lettuce wraps are a quick, easy, and nutritious option for a gastric bypass diet. They provide a balance of protein, healthy fats, and fiber to help keep you feeling full and satisfied.

29. Shrimp and avocado salad

Ingredients:

- 1 lb cooked shrimp, peeled and deveined
- 1 ripe avocado, diced
- 1 cup cherry tomatoes, halved
- 1/4 cup diced red onion
- 2 tbsp chopped fresh cilantro
- 2 tbsp lime juice
- 1 tbsp olive oil
- Salt and pepper to taste

Instructions:

1. In a large bowl, combine the cooked shrimp, diced avocado, cherry tomatoes, red onion, and cilantro.

2. In a small bowl, whisk together the lime juice and olive oil. Season with a pinch of salt and pepper.

3. Pour the dressing over the shrimp and avocado mixture and gently toss to coat.

4. Refrigerate for at least 30 minutes to allow the flavors to meld.

5. Serve chilled or at room temperature.

This shrimp and avocado salad is an excellent option for a gastric bypass diet. It's high in protein from the shrimp, healthy fats from the avocado, and low in carbs. The combination of lean protein, healthy fats, and fiber•rich vegetables makes it a satisfying and nutrient•dense meal.

Some tips:
- Use cooked, peeled, and deveined shrimp to save time.
- Adjust the portion size of shrimp and avocado to your individual needs.
- Add extra non•starchy vegetables, such as cucumber or bell pepper, for additional nutrients.
- This salad can be enjoyed on its own or served over a bed of mixed greens.

This shrimp and avocado salad is a great make•ahead option for a gastric bypass diet. It's easy to prepare, nutritious, and can be enjoyed as a main dish or a side.

30. Baked tilapia with asparagus

Ingredients:

- 4 (4 oz) tilapia fillets
- 1 tbsp olive oil
- 1 tsp lemon zest
- 1 tbsp lemon juice
- 1 tsp dried dill
- Salt and pepper to taste
- 1 lb asparagus, trimmed
- 1 tbsp grated Parmesan cheese (optional)

Instructions:

1. Preheat your oven to 400°F (200°C).

2. Place the tilapia fillets in a baking dish. Drizzle with the olive oil and sprinkle with the lemon zest, lemon juice, dried dill, salt, and pepper. Gently rub the seasoning into the fish.

3. Arrange the trimmed asparagus spears around the tilapia fillets in the baking dish.

4. Bake for 12•15 minutes, or until the tilapia is cooked through and flakes easily with a fork, and the asparagus is tender•crisp.

5. Remove the baked tilapia and asparagus from the oven. Sprinkle the Parmesan cheese over the asparagus, if desired.

6. Serve the baked tilapia and asparagus immediately.

This baked tilapia with asparagus is an excellent option for a gastric bypass diet. Tilapia is a lean, mild•flavored fish that is high in protein, while the asparagus provides fiber, vitamins, and minerals. The simple preparation and low•calorie ingredients make this a nutritious and satisfying meal.

Some tips:
- Choose fresh or frozen tilapia fillets for this recipe.
- Adjust the portion size of tilapia and asparagus to your individual needs.
- Experiment with different herbs and spices to add flavor without adding extra calories.
- Serve the baked tilapia and asparagus with a small portion of a low•carb vegetable side, such as roasted cauliflower or a side salad.

This baked tilapia with asparagus is a quick, easy, and nutritious meal option for a gastric bypass diet. It's a great way to incorporate lean protein and fiber•rich vegetables into your daily routine.

31. Baked salmon with roasted Brussels sprouts

Ingredients:

- 4 (4 oz) salmon fillets
- 1 tbsp olive oil
- 1 tsp lemon zest
- 1 tbsp lemon juice
- 1 tsp Dijon mustard
- Salt and pepper to taste
- 1 lb Brussels sprouts, trimmed and halved
- 1 tbsp olive oil
- 1 tsp garlic powder
- Salt and pepper to taste

Instructions:

1. Preheat your oven to 400°F (200°C).

2. In a small bowl, combine the olive oil, lemon zest, lemon juice, and Dijon mustard. Season the salmon fillets with salt and pepper, then brush the top of each fillet with the lemon•mustard mixture.

3. Place the salmon fillets in a baking dish and set aside.

4. In a separate baking dish, toss the trimmed and halved Brussels sprouts with the olive oil, garlic powder, salt, and pepper.

5. Roast the salmon and Brussels sprouts in the preheated oven for 15•20 minutes, or until the salmon is cooked through and flakes easily with a fork, and the Brussels sprouts are tender and lightly browned. Remove the baked salmon and roasted Brussels sprouts from the oven and serve immediately.

This baked salmon with roasted Brussels sprouts is an excellent option for a gastric bypass diet. Salmon is a rich source of lean protein and healthy omega•3 fatty acids, while the Brussels sprouts provide fiber, vitamins, and minerals. The simple preparation and nutrient•dense ingredients make this a satisfying and nutritious meal.

Some tips:
- Choose fresh or frozen salmon fillets for this recipe.
- Adjust the portion size of salmon and Brussels sprouts to your individual needs.
- Experiment with different seasonings, such as herbs or spices, to add flavor without adding extra calories.

32. Lean beef stir•fry with vegetables

Ingredients:

- 1 lb lean beef (such as sirloin or flank steak), thinly sliced
- 2 tbsp low•sodium soy sauce
- 1 tbsp rice vinegar
- 1 tsp sesame oil
- 1 tsp grated ginger
- 2 cloves garlic, minced
- 2 cups mixed vegetables (such as broccoli, bell peppers, snap peas, mushrooms)
- 1 tbsp olive oil
- Salt and pepper to taste

Instructions:

1. In a bowl, combine the sliced beef, soy sauce, rice vinegar, sesame oil, ginger, and garlic. Toss to coat the beef and let marinate for 15•20 minutes.

2. Heat the olive oil in a large skillet or wok over high heat.

3. Add the marinated beef and stir•fry for 2•3 minutes, until the beef is lightly browned but still pink in the center.

4. Add the mixed vegetables to the skillet and continue to stir•fry for 3•5 minutes, until the vegetables are tender•crisp.

5. Season with salt and pepper to taste.

6. Serve immediately, over a small portion of steamed cauliflower rice or zucchini noodles if desired.

Nutrition Information (per serving):
- Calories: 250•300
- Protein: 25•30g
- Fat: 10•15g
- Carbs: 10•15g
- Fiber: 4•6g

This lean beef and veggie stir•fry is packed with protein, fiber, and essential vitamins and minerals. The small portion size and focus on lean protein and non•starchy vegetables make it a great gastric bypass•friendly meal. Adjust the portion sizes as needed to fit your individual dietary needs.

33. Turkey meatballs with zucchini noodles

Ingredients:

- 1 lb ground turkey
- 1/4 cup almond flour
- 1 egg
- 2 tbsp grated Parmesan cheese
- 2 cloves garlic, minced
- 1 tsp dried oregano
- 1/2 tsp salt
- 1/4 tsp black pepper
- 2 medium zucchinis, spiralized or julienned into noodles
- 1 cup marinara sauce (low•sugar or no•sugar•added)
- 2 tbsp chopped fresh basil (optional)

Instructions:

1. Preheat your oven to 400°F (200°C).

2. In a large bowl, combine the ground turkey, almond flour, egg, Parmesan cheese, garlic, oregano, salt, and pepper. Mix well until the ingredients are fully incorporated.

3. Roll the turkey mixture into 1•inch meatballs and place them on a baking sheet lined with parchment paper.

4. Bake the turkey meatballs in the preheated oven for 18•20 minutes, or until they are cooked through and no longer pink in the center.

5. While the meatballs are baking, prepare the zucchini noodles. Use a spiralizer, julienne peeler, or mandoline slicer to cut the zucchinis into noodle•like strands.

6. In a large skillet, heat the marinara sauce over medium heat. Add the zucchini noodles and toss to coat them in the sauce. Cook for 2•3 minutes, just until the zucchini noodles are slightly softened.

7. Serve the turkey meatballs over the zucchini noodles, garnished with chopped fresh basil if desired.

This turkey meatballs with zucchini noodles dish is an excellent option for a gastric bypass diet. The turkey meatballs provide lean protein, while the zucchini noodles offer a low•carb, fiber•rich alternative to traditional pasta. The simple preparation and nutrient•dense ingredients make this a satisfying and nutritious meal.

34. Grilled chicken with quinoa and roasted vegetables

Ingredients:

- 4 (4 oz) boneless, skinless chicken breasts
- 1 tbsp olive oil
- 1 tsp dried oregano
- Salt and pepper to taste
- 1 cup uncooked quinoa, rinsed
- 2 cups low•sodium chicken broth
- 1 lb mixed vegetables (such as broccoli, bell peppers, zucchini), cut into 1•inch pieces
- 1 tbsp olive oil
- 1 tsp garlic powder
- Salt and pepper to taste

Instructions:

1. Preheat your grill or grill pan to medium•high heat.

2. Brush the chicken breasts with the olive oil and season with the dried oregano, salt, and pepper.

3. Grill the chicken for 4•6 minutes per side, or until it reaches an internal temperature of 165°F. Remove the grilled chicken from the heat and let it rest for a few minutes.

4. While the chicken is grilling, prepare the quinoa. In a medium saucepan, combine the rinsed quinoa and chicken broth. Bring the mixture to a boil, then reduce the heat to low, cover, and simmer for 15•20 minutes, until the quinoa is tender and the liquid is absorbed.

5. Preheat your oven to 400°F (200°C).

6. On a large baking sheet, toss the mixed vegetables with the olive oil, garlic powder, salt, and pepper.

7. Roast the vegetables in the preheated oven for 15•20 minutes, or until they are tender and lightly browned.

8. Serve the grilled chicken alongside the cooked quinoa and roasted vegetables.

This grilled chicken with quinoa and roasted vegetables is an excellent option for a gastric bypass diet. It's high in protein from the chicken, provides complex carbohydrates from the quinoa, and is packed with fiber•rich vegetables. The combination of lean protein, whole grains, and non•starchy vegetables makes it a satisfying and nutrient•dense meal.

35. Pork tenderloin with green beans

Ingredients:

- 1 lb pork tenderloin, trimmed of any visible fat
- 1 tbsp olive oil
- 1 tsp garlic powder
- 1 tsp dried thyme
- Salt and pepper to taste
- 1 lb fresh green beans, trimmed
- 1 tbsp olive oil
- 2 cloves garlic, minced
- 1/4 cup low•sodium chicken or vegetable broth

Instructions:

1. Preheat your oven to 400°F (200°C).

2. In a small bowl, combine the olive oil, garlic powder, dried thyme, salt, and pepper. Rub the seasoning mixture all over the pork tenderloin.

3. Place the seasoned pork tenderloin in a baking dish and roast in the preheated oven for 20•25 minutes, or until the internal temperature reaches 145°F.

4. While the pork is roasting, prepare the green beans. In a large skillet, heat the olive oil over medium•high heat.

5. Add the minced garlic to the skillet and sauté for 1 minute, until fragrant.

6. Add the trimmed green beans and the low•sodium broth to the skillet. Cover and cook for 5•7 minutes, stirring occasionally, until the green beans are tender•crisp.

7. Remove the pork tenderloin from the oven and let it rest for 5 minutes before slicing.

8. Serve the sliced pork tenderloin alongside the sautéed green beans.

This pork tenderloin with green beans is an excellent option for a gastric bypass diet. Pork tenderloin is a lean, high•protein protein source, while the green beans provide fiber and essential vitamins and minerals. The simple preparation and balance of macronutrients make this a satisfying and nutritious meal.

36. Tofu and vegetable curry

Ingredients:

- 1 block (14 oz) extra•firm tofu, cubed
- 1 tbsp olive oil
- 1 onion, diced
- 3 cloves garlic, minced
- 1 tbsp grated fresh ginger
- 2 tsp curry powder
- 1 tsp ground cumin
- 1 tsp ground coriander
- 1 can (13.5 oz) light coconut milk
- 1 cup low•sodium vegetable broth
- 2 cups mixed vegetables (such as cauliflower, bell peppers, spinach)
- 1 tbsp lime juice
- Salt and pepper to taste
- Chopped fresh cilantro for garnish (optional)

Instructions:

1. In a large skillet or wok, heat the olive oil over medium•high heat.

2. Add the cubed tofu and sauté for 3•4 minutes, until lightly browned on all sides. Remove the tofu from the skillet and set it aside.

3. In the same skillet, sauté the diced onion for 2•3 minutes, until translucent.

4. Add the minced garlic and grated ginger to the skillet and cook for 1 minute, until fragrant.

5. Stir in the curry powder, cumin, and coriander. Cook for 1 minute to toast the spices.

6. Pour in the coconut milk and vegetable broth. Bring the mixture to a simmer.

7. Add the mixed vegetables to the skillet and cook for 5•7 minutes, until the vegetables are tender•crisp.

8. Stir the sautéed tofu back into the curry and add the lime juice. Season with salt and pepper to taste. Serve the tofu and vegetable curry warm, garnished with chopped fresh cilantro if desired.

This tofu and vegetable curry is a delicious and nutritious meal option for a gastric bypass diet. It's a great way to incorporate plant•based protein, healthy fats, and fiber•rich vegetables into your daily routine.

37. Baked cod with sautéed spinach

Ingredients:

- 4 cod fillets (about 1 lb total)
- 2 tbsp olive oil
- 1 tsp paprika
- Salt and pepper to taste
- 1 lb fresh spinach, washed and stems removed
- 2 cloves garlic, minced
- 1 tbsp lemon juice

Instructions:

1. Preheat oven to 400°F. Line a baking sheet with parchment paper.

2. Place the cod fillets on the prepared baking sheet. Drizzle with 1 tbsp of the olive oil and sprinkle with paprika, salt, and pepper.

3. Bake for 12•15 minutes, until the cod is opaque and flakes easily with a fork.

4. While the cod is baking, heat the remaining 1 tbsp of olive oil in a large skillet over medium heat. Add the garlic and cook for 1 minute until fragrant.

5. Add the spinach to the skillet and sauté for 2•3 minutes, until the spinach is wilted.

6. Remove the skillet from heat and stir in the lemon juice. Season with salt and pepper to taste.

7. Serve the baked cod immediately, topped with the sautéed spinach.

Enjoy your healthy and delicious baked cod with sautéed spinach!

38. Chicken and cauliflower rice bowl

Ingredients:

- 1 lb boneless, skinless chicken breasts, cubed
- 1 tbsp olive oil
- 1 tsp garlic powder
- 1 tsp onion powder
- Salt and pepper to taste
- 4 cups riced cauliflower (or 1 head of cauliflower, riced)
- 1 cup diced bell peppers
- 1/2 cup diced onion
- 2 tbsp low•sodium soy sauce or tamari
- 1 tbsp rice vinegar
- 1 tsp sesame oil
- Chopped fresh cilantro for garnish (optional)

Instructions:

1. Preheat your oven to 400°F (200°C).

2. In a large bowl, toss the cubed chicken with the olive oil, garlic powder, onion powder, salt, and pepper.

3. Spread the seasoned chicken on a baking sheet and roast in the preheated oven for 15•20 minutes, or until the chicken is cooked through and no longer pink.

4. While the chicken is baking, prepare the cauliflower rice. If using a whole head of cauliflower, grate or pulse it in a food processor until it resembles rice•sized grains.

5. In a large skillet or wok, sauté the diced bell peppers and onion over medium•high heat for 3•4 minutes, until they start to soften.

6. Add the riced cauliflower to the skillet and continue to sauté for 5•7 minutes, stirring frequently, until the cauliflower is tender.

7. Stir in the cooked chicken, soy sauce or tamari, rice vinegar, and sesame oil. Toss to combine. Serve the chicken and cauliflower rice bowl warm, garnished with chopped fresh cilantro if desired.

This chicken and cauliflower rice bowl is an excellent option for a gastric bypass diet. It's high in protein from the chicken, low in carbs thanks to the cauliflower rice, and packed with fiber•rich vegetables. The combination of lean protein, healthy fats, and non•starchy vegetables makes it a satisfying and nutrient•dense meal.

39. Seared scallops with a side of mixed greens

Ingredients:

- 1 lb sea scallops, patted dry
- 1 tbsp olive oil
- Salt and pepper to taste
- 4 cups mixed greens (such as spinach, arugula, kale)
- 1 tbsp olive oil
- 1 tbsp lemon juice
- 1 tsp Dijon mustard
- Salt and pepper to taste

Instructions:

1. Heat a large skillet over high heat. Add the olive oil.

2. Season the scallops with salt and pepper on both sides.

3. Sear the scallops in the hot skillet for 2•3 minutes per side, until they are golden brown and cooked through. Be careful not to overcrowd the pan.

4. Remove the seared scallops from the skillet and set them aside.

5. In a large bowl, combine the mixed greens.

6. In a small bowl, whisk together the olive oil, lemon juice, and Dijon mustard. Season the dressing with salt and pepper to taste.

7. Drizzle the dressing over the mixed greens and toss to coat. Divide the mixed greens salad onto plates and top with the seared scallops.

Nutrition Information (per serving):
- Calories: 250•300
- Protein: 25•30g
- Fat: 12•15g
- Carbs: 5•10g
- Fiber: 2•3g

This seared scallops with mixed greens dish is an excellent option for a gastric bypass diet. Scallops are a lean, high•protein seafood, while the mixed greens provide a nutrient•dense, low•carb side. The simple preparation and balance of macronutrients make this a satisfying and healthy meal.

40. Beef and broccoli stir•fry

Ingredients:

- 1 lb flank steak or sirloin, thinly sliced
- 2 tbsp low•sodium soy sauce
- 1 tbsp rice vinegar
- 1 tsp sesame oil
- 2 tsp grated ginger
- 2 cloves garlic, minced
- 2 cups broccoli florets
- 1 tbsp olive oil
- Salt and pepper to taste

Instructions:

1. In a bowl, combine the sliced beef, soy sauce, rice vinegar, sesame oil, ginger, and garlic. Toss to coat the beef and let it marinate for 15•20 minutes.

2. Heat the olive oil in a large skillet or wok over high heat.

3. Add the marinated beef and stir•fry for 2•3 minutes, until the beef is lightly browned but still pink in the center.

4. Add the broccoli florets to the skillet and continue to stir•fry for 3•5 minutes, until the broccoli is tender•crisp.

5. Season the beef and broccoli with salt and pepper to taste.

6. Serve the beef and broccoli stir•fry immediately.

Nutrition Information (per serving):
- Calories: 250•300
- Protein: 30•35g
- Fat: 10•12g
- Carbs: 10•15g
- Fiber: 4•6g

This beef and broccoli stir•fry is an excellent option for a gastric bypass diet. It's high in protein from the lean beef, low in carbs, and packed with fiber•rich broccoli. The simple preparation and nutrient•dense ingredients make it a satisfying and nutritious meal.

41. Protein mug cake

Ingredients:

- 2 tbsp whey protein powder (unflavored or vanilla)
- 1 tbsp ground flaxseed
- 1 tbsp granulated erythritol or other low•calorie sweetener
- 1 egg
- 2 tbsp unsweetened almond milk
- 1/4 tsp baking powder
- 1/4 tsp vanilla extract (optional)

Instructions:

1. In a microwave•safe mug or ramekin, whisk together the protein powder, flaxseed, and sweetener.

2. Add the egg and almond milk, and stir until well combined.

3. Stir in the baking powder and vanilla extract (if using).

4. Microwave the mug cake for 60•90 seconds, until it is set in the center.

5. Allow the mug cake to cool for 1•2 minutes before enjoying.

Optional Toppings:
- A drizzle of sugar•free syrup or melted sugar•free chocolate
- Fresh berries
- A sprinkle of cinnamon or nutmeg

Notes:
- Use a whey protein powder that is unflavored or vanilla•flavored for best results.
- Erythritol is a zero•calorie sweetener that works well in this recipe, but you can use other low•calorie sweeteners like stevia or monk fruit if preferred.
- The ground flaxseed adds fiber and healthy fats to the mug cake.
- Be careful not to overcook, as the mug cake can become dry.

This high protein mug cake is a great option for those following a gastric bypass diet, as it is low in calories and carbs but high in protein to help meet nutritional needs. Enjoy it as a quick and satisfying snack or dessert!

42. Greek yogurt with honey and nuts

Ingredients:

- 1 cup plain Greek yogurt
- 2 tbsp honey
- 2 tbsp chopped nuts (such as almonds, walnuts, or pecans)

Instructions:

1. Scoop the Greek yogurt into a serving bowl.

2. Drizzle the honey over the top of the yogurt.

3. Sprinkle the chopped nuts over the honey.

4. Gently stir the honey and nuts into the yogurt until well combined.

5. Serve immediately.

Optional Variations:
- Top with fresh berries like blueberries, raspberries, or sliced strawberries.
- Add a sprinkle of cinnamon or vanilla extract.
- Use a flavored Greek yogurt instead of plain.
- Substitute maple syrup or agave nectar for the honey.

This simple Greek yogurt parfait makes a delicious and healthy breakfast, snack, or light dessert. The combination of creamy yogurt, sweet honey, and crunchy nuts is both satisfying and nutritious. Enjoy!

43. Cottage cheese with a drizzle of honey

Ingredients:

- 1 cup low•fat or non•fat cottage cheese
- 1•2 tablespoons honey

Instructions:

1. Scoop the cottage cheese into a small bowl.

2. Drizzle the honey over the top of the cottage cheese.

3. Gently stir the honey into the cottage cheese until it is evenly distributed.

4. Serve immediately.

Optional Variations:

- Top with fresh fruit like berries, sliced peaches, or diced mango

- Sprinkle with a pinch of cinnamon or nutmeg.

- Add a tablespoon of chopped nuts like almonds, walnuts, or pecans.

- Use a flavored honey like lavender or wildflower.

This simple cottage cheese and honey dish makes a great healthy snack or light breakfast. The protein•rich cottage cheese paired with the natural sweetness of honey is a delicious and satisfying combination.

For those following a gastric bypass diet, this recipe is a great option as it is low in calories and easy to digest. The cottage cheese provides important nutrients like calcium and protein, while the honey adds a touch of sweetness without too many carbs.

Enjoy this simple yet flavorful cottage cheese and honey treat!

44. Protein ice cream

Ingredients:

- 1 cup plain Greek yogurt
- 1/2 cup unsweetened almond milk
- 1/4 cup whey protein powder
- 2 tbsp granulated erythritol or other low•calorie sweetener
- 1 tsp vanilla extract
- 1/4 tsp xanthan gum (optional, for thicker texture)

Instructions:

1. In a medium bowl, whisk together the Greek yogurt, almond milk, protein powder, erythritol, and vanilla extract until well combined.

2. If using xanthan gum, sprinkle it over the mixture and whisk vigorously to incorporate.

3. Pour the mixture into an ice cream maker and churn according to manufacturer's instructions, usually 20•30 minutes.

4. Transfer the churned ice cream to an airtight container and freeze for at least 2 hours before serving.

5. Scoop and serve the protein ice cream.

Notes:

- Use a whey protein powder that is unflavored or vanilla•flavored for best results.

- Erythritol is a zero•calorie sweetener that works well in this recipe, but you can use other low•calorie sweeteners like stevia or monk fruit if preferred.

- For a creamier texture, you can add 1•2 tbsp of heavy cream or full•fat coconut milk to the mixture.

- Top with fresh berries, chopped nuts, or a drizzle of sugar•free chocolate sauce.

This high protein ice cream is a great option for those following a gastric bypass diet, as it's low in sugar and calories but high in protein to help meet nutritional needs. Enjoy!

45. Chia seed pudding

Ingredients:

- 1/4 cup chia seeds
- 1 cup unsweetened almond milk (or other non•dairy milk)
- 1 tbsp honey or maple syrup (optional)
- 1/2 tsp vanilla extract
- 1/4 tsp ground cinnamon (optional)
- Fresh berries or sliced almonds for topping (optional)

Instructions:

1. In a medium bowl, whisk together the chia seeds, almond milk, honey or maple syrup (if using), vanilla extract, and cinnamon (if using) until well combined.

2. Cover the bowl and refrigerate for at least 2 hours, or overnight, stirring occasionally, until the chia seeds have thickened the mixture into a pudding•like consistency.

3. Divide the chia seed pudding into individual serving bowls or containers.

4. Top the chia seed pudding with fresh berries, sliced almonds, or any other desired toppings.

5. Serve chilled.

This chia seed pudding is an excellent option for a gastric bypass diet. Chia seeds are high in protein, fiber, and healthy omega•3 fatty acids, making them a nutrient•dense ingredient. The pudding is low in carbs and can be customized with various toppings to suit your taste preferences.

Some tips:
- Use unsweetened almond milk or another non•dairy milk to keep the calorie and sugar content low.
- Add a small amount of honey or maple syrup if you prefer a slightly sweeter pudding.
- Top the pudding with fresh berries, sliced almonds, or other low•carb toppings for added flavor and nutrients.
- Adjust the portion size to your individual needs, as a 1/2 cup serving can be a satisfying snack or light meal.
- Prepare the chia seed pudding in advance and store it in the refrigerator for easy access throughout the week.

This chia seed pudding is a versatile, nutrient•dense, and easy•to•prepare option for a gastric bypass diet. It's a great way to incorporate healthy fats, protein, and fiber into your daily routine.

46. High•protein cheesecake

Ingredients:

- 1 cup almond flour
- 2 tbsp granulated erythritol or other low•calorie sweetener
- 2 tbsp unsalted butter, melted

Filling:
- 24 oz (3 packages) low•fat cream cheese, softened
- 1 cup plain Greek yogurt
- 1/2 cup granulated erythritol or other low•calorie sweetener
- 2 scoops (about 1/2 cup) vanilla protein powder
- 2 eggs
- 1 tsp vanilla extract
- 1/4 tsp salt

Instructions:

1. Preheat oven to 325°F (165°C). Grease a 9•inch springform pan.

Crust:
2. In a medium bowl, mix together the almond flour, erythritol, and melted butter until well combined. Press the mixture evenly into the bottom of the prepared springform pan.

Filling:
4. In a large bowl, beat the cream cheese with an electric mixer until smooth and creamy.

5. Add the Greek yogurt, erythritol, protein powder, eggs, vanilla, and salt. Beat until well incorporated and smooth.

6. Pour the cheesecake batter over the prepared crust.

7. Bake for 45•55 minutes, until the center is almost set. The cheesecake should still have a slight jiggle in the center.

8. Turn off the oven and leave the cheesecake inside with the door closed for 1 hour.

9. Remove the cheesecake from the oven and allow it to cool completely at room temperature, then refrigerate for at least 4 hours or overnight before serving.

This high•protein cheesecake is a delicious and satisfying treat that is suitable for those following a gastric bypass diet. The combination of low•fat cream cheese, Greek yogurt, and protein powder provides a boost of protein while keeping the carbs and sugar low.

47. Almond flour cookies

Ingredients:

- 2 cups almond flour
- 1/4 cup granulated erythritol or other low•calorie sweetener
- 1/4 tsp salt
- 1/2 tsp baking soda
- 1/2 cup unsalted butter, softened
- 1 egg
- 1 tsp vanilla extract

Instructions:

1. Preheat your oven to 350°F (175°C). Line a baking sheet with parchment paper.

2. In a medium bowl, whisk together the almond flour, erythritol, salt, and baking soda.

3. In a separate large bowl, beat the softened butter with an electric mixer until creamy. Add the egg and vanilla extract, and beat until well combined.

4. Gradually add the dry ingredients to the wet ingredients, mixing until a dough forms.

5. Scoop the dough by the tablespoonful and place them about 2 inches apart on the prepared baking sheet.

6. Bake for 10•12 minutes, or until the cookies are lightly golden around the edges.

7. Allow the cookies to cool on the baking sheet for 5 minutes before transferring them to a wire rack to cool completely.

Optional Variations:
- Add 1/4 cup of chopped nuts or sugar•free chocolate chips to the dough.
- Sprinkle the cookies with a pinch of cinnamon or nutmeg before baking.
- Dip the cooled cookies in melted sugar•free chocolate.

These almond flour cookies are a great option for those following a gastric bypass diet. They are low in carbs, high in healthy fats from the almond flour, and provide a satisfying cookie•like treat. Enjoy them as a snack or light dessert.

Remember to adjust the serving size as needed to fit your dietary needs. Savor these delicious and nutritious almond flour cookies!

48. Low•sugar protein brownies

Ingredients:

- 1/2 cup unsweetened applesauce
- 1/4 cup unsweetened cocoa powder
- 1/4 cup whey protein powder (unflavored or chocolate)
- 2 tbsp granulated erythritol or other low•calorie sweetener
- 1 egg
- 1 tsp vanilla extract
- 1/4 tsp baking powder
- Pinch of salt

Instructions:

1. Preheat your oven to 350°F (175°C). Grease an 8x8 inch baking pan or line it with parchment paper.

2. In a medium bowl, whisk together the applesauce, cocoa powder, protein powder, erythritol, egg, vanilla, baking powder, and salt until well combined.

3. Pour the batter into the prepared baking pan and spread it out evenly.

4. Bake for 18•22 minutes, or until a toothpick inserted in the center comes out clean.

5. Allow the brownies to cool completely in the pan before cutting into squares.

Optional Toppings:
- Chopped nuts (such as walnuts or pecans)
- A drizzle of sugar•free chocolate sauce
- Fresh berries

Notes:
- Use an unflavored or chocolate•flavored whey protein powder for best results.
- Erythritol is a zero•calorie sweetener that works well in this recipe, but you can use other low•calorie sweeteners like stevia or monk fruit if preferred.
- The applesauce helps keep the brownies moist without adding too much sugar.
- Be careful not to overbake, as the brownies can become dry.

These low•sugar, high protein brownies are a great option for those following a gastric bypass diet. They provide a satisfying chocolate treat while being low in carbs and high in protein to support your nutritional needs. Enjoy!

49. Ricotta cheese with berries

Ingredients:

- 1/2 cup low•fat or non•fat ricotta cheese
- 1/4 cup fresh berries (such as blueberries, raspberries, or blackberries)
- 1 tsp honey or sugar•free syrup (optional)
- Cinnamon (optional)

Instructions:

1. Scoop the ricotta cheese into a small bowl.

2. Gently fold in the fresh berries until they are evenly distributed throughout the ricotta.

3. If desired, drizzle the honey or sugar•free syrup over the top of the ricotta and berries.

4. Sprinkle a light dusting of cinnamon over the top (optional).

5. Serve immediately.

Notes:
- Use low•fat or non•fat ricotta cheese to keep the calorie and fat content low.

- Choose fresh, in•season berries for maximum flavor and nutrition.

- The honey or sugar•free syrup is optional, as the berries provide natural sweetness.

- Cinnamon adds a warm, comforting flavor without any additional calories or sugar.

This simple ricotta and berry dish is a great option for those following a gastric bypass diet. The ricotta provides a good source of protein, while the berries offer fiber, vitamins, and antioxidants. It makes a satisfying and nutritious snack or light dessert.

Feel free to experiment with different berry combinations or add a sprinkle of chopped nuts for some extra crunch. Enjoy this delicious and healthy treat!

50. Protein•infused chocolate mousse

Ingredients:

- 1 cup plain Greek yogurt
- 1/4 cup unsweetened cocoa powder
- 2 scoops (about 1/2 cup) chocolate protein powder
- 2 tbsp granulated erythritol or other low•calorie sweetener
- 1 tsp vanilla extract
- Pinch of salt

Instructions:

1. In a medium bowl, whisk together the Greek yogurt, cocoa powder, protein powder, erythritol, vanilla, and salt until well combined and smooth.

2. Divide the chocolate mousse mixture evenly between 4 small ramekins or serving dishes.

3. Cover and refrigerate for at least 2 hours, or until set.

Optional Toppings:
- Fresh berries (such as raspberries or strawberries)
- Shaved dark chocolate
- Chopped nuts (such as almonds or walnuts)
- A drizzle of sugar•free chocolate sauce

Notes:
- Use a high•quality, unsweetened cocoa powder for the best chocolate flavor.

- Choose a chocolate•flavored whey or casein protein powder for this recipe.

- Erythritol is a zero•calorie sweetener that works well in this recipe, but you can use other low•calorie sweeteners like stevia or monk fruit if preferred.

- The Greek yogurt provides a creamy, protein•rich base for the mousse. Adjust the sweetener to your personal taste preference.

This protein•infused chocolate mousse is a delicious and satisfying treat that is suitable for those following a gastric bypass diet. The combination of protein, healthy fats, and antioxidants from the cocoa powder makes it a nutritious dessert option.

Enjoy a small serving of this rich and creamy chocolate mousse as a special indulgence or a post•workout snack. Adjust the portion size as needed to fit your dietary needs.

51. Chicken and vegetable soup

Ingredients:

- 1 lb boneless, skinless chicken breasts, cubed
- 1 tbsp olive oil
- 1 onion, diced
- 3 carrots, peeled and sliced
- 3 celery stalks, sliced
- 3 cloves garlic, minced
- 6 cups low•sodium chicken broth
- 1 (14.5 oz) can diced tomatoes
- 1 cup frozen green beans
- 1 cup frozen peas
- 1 tsp dried thyme
- 1 tsp dried oregano
- Salt and pepper to taste
- Chopped parsley for garnish (optional)

Instructions:

1. In a large pot or Dutch oven, heat the olive oil over medium heat. Add the cubed chicken and cook for 3•4 minutes, until lightly browned.

2. Add the onion, carrots, celery, and garlic. Sauté for 5•7 minutes, until the vegetables start to soften.

3. Pour in the chicken broth and diced tomatoes. Stir in the green beans, peas, thyme, and oregano. Season with salt and pepper to taste.

4. Bring the soup to a boil, then reduce heat and let it simmer for 20•25 minutes, or until the chicken is cooked through and the vegetables are tender.

5. Taste and adjust seasoning as needed.

6. Ladle the chicken and vegetable soup into bowls and garnish with chopped parsley, if desired.

Serve hot, with crusty bread or a side salad.

This chicken and vegetable soup is a nutritious and filling option for those following a gastric bypass diet. The combination of lean protein, fiber•rich vegetables, and low•sodium broth makes it a great choice for a satisfying and healthy meal.

52. Lentil soup

Ingredients:

- 1 tbsp olive oil
- 1 onion, diced
- 3 cloves garlic, minced
- 2 carrots, peeled and diced
- 2 celery stalks, diced
- 1 cup dried brown or green lentils, rinsed
- 6 cups low•sodium vegetable or chicken broth
- 1 (14.5 oz) can diced tomatoes
- 1 tsp dried thyme
- 1 tsp dried oregano
- Salt and pepper to taste
- Chopped parsley for garnish (optional)

Instructions:

1. In a large pot or Dutch oven, heat the olive oil over medium heat. Add the onion and sauté for 3•4 minutes until translucent.

2. Add the garlic, carrots, and celery. Sauté for another 2•3 minutes until fragrant.

3. Stir in the lentils, broth, diced tomatoes, thyme, and oregano. Season with salt and pepper to taste.

4. Bring the soup to a boil, then reduce heat and let it simmer for 20•25 minutes, or until the lentils are tender.

5. Taste and adjust seasoning as needed.

6. Ladle the lentil soup into bowls and garnish with chopped parsley if desired.

Serve hot, with crusty bread or a side salad.

Notes:
- For a creamier texture, you can blend a portion of the soup using an immersion blender.
- Add diced potatoes, spinach, or kale for extra nutrition.
- Use low•sodium broth to keep the sodium content down.
- This soup freezes well for easy meal prep.

53. Beef and vegetable stew

Ingredients:

- 1 lb beef stew meat, cut into 1•inch cubes
- 2 tbsp olive oil
- 1 onion, diced
- 3 carrots, peeled and diced
- 3 celery stalks, diced
- 3 cloves garlic, minced
- 4 cups low•sodium beef or chicken broth
- 1 (14.5 oz) can diced tomatoes
- 2 medium potatoes, peeled and diced
- 1 cup frozen peas
- 1 tsp dried thyme
- 1 bay leaf
- Salt and pepper to taste
- Chopped parsley for garnish (optional)

Instructions:

1. In a large pot or Dutch oven, heat the olive oil over medium•high heat. Add the beef cubes and brown on all sides, about 5•7 minutes total. Remove the beef from the pot and set aside.

2. Reduce heat to medium, add the onion, carrots, celery, and garlic to the pot. Sauté for 5•7 minutes until the vegetables start to soften.

3. Pour in the broth and diced tomatoes. Add the browned beef, potatoes, peas, thyme, and bay leaf. Season with salt and pepper to taste.

4. Bring the stew to a boil, then reduce heat and let it simmer for 45•60 minutes, or until the beef and vegetables are very tender.

5. Remove the bay leaf. Taste and adjust seasoning as needed.

6. Ladle the beef and vegetable stew into bowls and garnish with chopped parsley, if desired.

Serve hot, with a side of crusty bread or a fresh salad.

This beef and vegetable stew is a hearty and nutritious option for those following a gastric bypass diet. The combination of lean protein, fiber•rich vegetables, and savory broth makes it a satisfying and filling meal. Enjoy!

54. Turkey and black bean soup

Ingredients:

- 1 tbsp olive oil
- 1 onion, diced
- 3 cloves garlic, minced
- 1 lb ground turkey
- 2 cans (15 oz each) black beans, rinsed and drained
- 1 can (14.5 oz) diced tomatoes
- 4 cups low•sodium chicken or vegetable broth
- 1 tsp ground cumin
- 1 tsp dried oregano
- 1/2 tsp chili powder
- Salt and pepper to taste
- Chopped cilantro for garnish (optional)

Instructions:

1. In a large pot or Dutch oven, heat the olive oil over medium heat. Add the onion and sauté for 3•4 minutes until translucent.

2. Add the garlic and ground turkey. Cook, breaking up the turkey with a wooden spoon, until the turkey is browned, about 5•7 minutes.

3. Stir in the black beans, diced tomatoes, broth, cumin, oregano, and chili powder. Season with salt and pepper to taste.

4. Bring the soup to a boil, then reduce heat and let it simmer for 20•25 minutes, stirring occasionally, until the flavors have melded and the soup has thickened slightly.

5. Taste and adjust seasoning as needed.

6. Ladle the turkey and black bean soup into bowls and garnish with chopped cilantro, if desired.

Serve hot, with a side of crusty bread or a fresh salad.

This turkey and black bean soup is a hearty and nutritious option for those following a gastric bypass diet. The combination of lean protein, fiber•rich beans, and flavorful spices makes it a satisfying and filling meal. Enjoy!

55. Split pea soup with ham

Ingredients:

- 1 tbsp olive oil
- 1 onion, diced
- 3 carrots, peeled and diced
- 3 celery stalks, diced
- 3 cloves garlic, minced
- 1 lb dried split peas, rinsed
- 6 cups low•sodium chicken or vegetable broth
- 1 cup diced cooked ham
- 1 bay leaf
- 1 tsp dried thyme
- Salt and pepper to taste

Instructions:

1. In a large pot or Dutch oven, heat the olive oil over medium heat. Add the onion, carrots, celery, and garlic. Sauté for 5•7 minutes until the vegetables start to soften.

2. Stir in the rinsed split peas, broth, diced ham, bay leaf, and thyme. Season with salt and pepper to taste.

3. Bring the soup to a boil, then reduce heat and let it simmer for 45•60 minutes, stirring occasionally, until the split peas are very soft and the soup has thickened.

4. Remove the bay leaf. Use an immersion blender or regular blender to puree about half of the soup, leaving some texture.

5. Taste and adjust seasoning as needed.

6. Ladle the split pea soup into bowls and serve hot.

Optional Garnishes:
- Chopped parsley or chives
- A drizzle of olive oil
- Croutons or crusty bread

Split pea soup is a hearty, protein•rich dish that is perfect for those following a gastric bypass diet. The combination of fiber•filled split peas and lean ham makes it a satisfying and nutritious meal.

Enjoy this comforting split pea soup on a chilly day or as part of a balanced meal. Adjust the portion size as needed to fit your dietary needs.

56. Seafood chowder

Ingredients:

- 1 tbsp olive oil
- 1 onion, diced
- 2 carrots, peeled and diced
- 2 celery stalks, diced
- 3 cloves garlic, minced
- 2 cups low•sodium chicken or vegetable broth
- 1 cup unsweetened almond milk
- 1 lb white fish fillets (such as cod, halibut, or tilapia), cut into 1•inch pieces
- 1 lb peeled and deveined shrimp
- 1 tsp dried thyme
- 1/2 tsp smoked paprika
- Salt and pepper to taste
- Chopped parsley for garnish (optional)

Instructions:

1. In a large pot or Dutch oven, heat the olive oil over medium heat. Add the onion, carrots, celery, and garlic. Sauté for 5•7 minutes until the vegetables start to soften.

2. Pour in the broth and almond milk. Bring the mixture to a simmer.

3. Add the white fish, shrimp, thyme, and smoked paprika. Season with salt and pepper to taste.

4. Reduce heat and let the chowder simmer for 15•20 minutes, or until the fish and shrimp are cooked through and the vegetables are tender.

5. Taste and adjust seasoning as needed. Ladle the seafood chowder into bowls and garnish with chopped parsley, if desired.

Notes:
- Use low•sodium broth to keep the sodium content down.
- For a creamier texture, you can blend a portion of the chowder using an immersion blender.
- Substitute other types of seafood, such as scallops or crab meat, if desired.
- Add diced potatoes or corn for extra heartiness.
- This chowder freezes well for easy meal prep.

This seafood chowder is a delicious and nutritious option for those following a gastric bypass diet. The combination of lean protein from the fish and shrimp, along with the creamy broth and vegetables, makes it a satisfying and filling meal. Enjoy!

57. Tomato basil soup with added protein powder

Ingredients:

- 1 tbsp olive oil
- 1 onion, diced
- 3 cloves garlic, minced
- 1 (28 oz) can crushed tomatoes
- 2 cups low•sodium chicken or vegetable broth
- 1/4 cup unflavored or vanilla protein powder
- 1/4 cup fresh basil leaves, chopped
- 1 tsp dried oregano
- Salt and pepper to taste
- Grated Parmesan cheese for serving (optional)

Instructions:

1. In a large pot or Dutch oven, heat the olive oil over medium heat. Add the onion and sauté for 3•4 minutes until translucent.

2. Add the garlic and sauté for 1 minute until fragrant.

3. Pour in the crushed tomatoes and broth. Whisk in the protein powder until fully incorporated.

4. Stir in the chopped basil and dried oregano. Season with salt and pepper to taste.

5. Bring the soup to a simmer and cook for 10•15 minutes, stirring occasionally, until slightly thickened.

6. Ladle the tomato basil protein soup into bowls. Top with a sprinkle of grated Parmesan cheese, if desired. Serve hot, with crusty bread or a side salad.

Notes:
- Use an unflavored or vanilla•flavored protein powder for the best flavor integration.
- Adjust the amount of protein powder to your desired thickness and protein content.
- For a creamier texture, you can blend a portion of the soup using an immersion blender.
- Add diced cooked chicken or turkey for extra protein.
- Garnish with fresh basil leaves, a drizzle of olive oil, or a sprinkle of red pepper flakes.

This tomato basil protein soup is a nutritious and satisfying option for those following a gastric bypass diet. The added protein powder boosts the protein content, while the tomatoes, basil, and broth provide a flavorful and comforting soup experience. Enjoy!

58. Mushroom and barley soup

Ingredients:

- 1 tbsp olive oil
- 1 onion, diced
- 3 cloves garlic, minced
- 8 oz cremini or button mushrooms, sliced
- 1 cup pearl barley, rinsed
- 6 cups low•sodium chicken or vegetable broth
- 1 tsp dried thyme
- 1 bay leaf
- Salt and pepper to taste
- Chopped parsley for garnish (optional)

Instructions:

1. In a large pot or Dutch oven, heat the olive oil over medium heat. Add the onion and sauté for 3•4 minutes until translucent.

2. Add the garlic and mushrooms. Sauté for an additional 5 minutes, until the mushrooms are softened.

3. Stir in the pearl barley, broth, thyme, and bay leaf. Season with salt and pepper to taste.

4. Bring the soup to a boil, then reduce heat and let it simmer for 30•40 minutes, or until the barley is tender.

5. Remove the bay leaf. Taste and adjust seasoning as needed. Ladle the mushroom and barley soup into bowls and garnish with chopped parsley, if desired.

Serve hot, with a side salad or a slice of whole•grain toast.

Notes:
- Use low•sodium broth to keep the sodium content down.
- For a creamier texture, you can blend a portion of the soup using an immersion blender.
- Add diced carrots, celery, or spinach for extra nutrition.
- This soup freezes well for easy meal prep.

The barley in this soup provides a good source of fiber, while the mushrooms and broth offer a savory, umami•rich flavor. This mushroom and barley soup is a hearty and satisfying option for those following a gastric bypass diet.

59. White bean and chicken chili

Ingredients:

- 1 tbsp olive oil
- 1 onion, diced
- 3 cloves garlic, minced
- 1 lb boneless, skinless chicken breasts, cubed
- 2 cans (15 oz each) white beans, rinsed and drained
- 4 cups low•sodium chicken broth
- 1 can (4 oz) diced green chiles
- 1 tsp ground cumin
- 1 tsp dried oregano
- 1/2 tsp chili powder
- Salt and pepper to taste
- Chopped cilantro for garnish (optional)

Instructions:

1. In a large pot or Dutch oven, heat the olive oil over medium heat. Add the onion and sauté for 3•4 minutes until translucent.

2. Add the garlic and chicken. Cook, stirring occasionally, until the chicken is lightly browned, about 5•7 minutes.

3. Stir in the white beans, chicken broth, diced green chiles, cumin, oregano, and chili powder. Season with salt and pepper to taste.

4. Bring the chili to a boil, then reduce heat and let it simmer for 20•25 minutes, stirring occasionally, until the chicken is cooked through and the flavors have melded.

5. Taste and adjust seasoning as needed. Ladle the white bean and chicken chili into bowls and garnish with chopped cilantro, if desired.

Serve hot, with a side of steamed cauliflower or a fresh salad.

Notes:
- Use low•sodium chicken broth to keep the sodium content down.
- For a creamier texture, you can blend a portion of the chili using an immersion blender.
- Add diced avocado or a sprinkle of shredded cheese as a topping, if desired.
- This chili freezes well for easy meal prep.

This white bean and chicken chili is a hearty and protein•packed option for those following a gastric bypass diet. The combination of lean chicken, fiber•rich beans, and flavorful spices makes it a satisfying and nutritious meal. Enjoy!

60. Miso soup with tofu

Ingredients:

- 4 cups low•sodium vegetable or chicken broth
- 2 tbsp white or yellow miso paste
- 1 block (14 oz) firm or extra•firm tofu, cubed
- 1 cup sliced mushrooms (such as shiitake or cremini)
- 2 cups baby spinach or kale, chopped
- 2 green onions, sliced
- 1 tsp sesame oil (optional)

Instructions:

1. In a medium saucepan, bring the broth to a gentle simmer over medium heat.

2. In a small bowl, whisk together the miso paste with a few tablespoons of the hot broth until smooth.

3. Carefully pour the miso mixture back into the saucepan with the remaining broth, whisking to combine.

4. Add the cubed tofu, mushrooms, and spinach or kale to the broth. Simmer for 3•5 minutes, until the greens are wilted and the tofu is heated through.

5. Remove the saucepan from heat and stir in the sliced green onions.

6. Drizzle with sesame oil, if desired.

7. Ladle the miso soup into bowls and serve immediately.

Notes:
- Use low•sodium broth to keep the sodium content down.
- Adjust the amount of miso paste to your taste preference.
- Feel free to add other vegetables like carrots, daikon, or bok choy.
- For a heartier meal, serve the miso soup with a side of steamed brown rice or quinoa.

This miso soup with tofu is a nourishing and comforting option for those following a gastric bypass diet. The miso paste provides a savory, umami•rich flavor, while the tofu and vegetables offer a good source of protein, fiber, and essential nutrients.

Enjoy this simple yet satisfying miso soup as a light meal or appetizer. Adjust the portion size as needed to fit your dietary needs.

61. Shrimp cocktail

Ingredients:

- 1 lb cooked and chilled shrimp, peeled and deveined
- 1/2 cup low•sugar cocktail sauce
- 1 lemon, cut into wedges
- Chopped parsley for garnish (optional)

Instructions:

1. Arrange the cooked shrimp on a serving platter or in individual cocktail glasses.

2. Serve the shrimp with the low•sugar cocktail sauce on the side for dipping.

3. Garnish with lemon wedges and chopped parsley, if desired.

Tips:
- Use large or jumbo shrimp for a more impressive presentation.

- For the cocktail sauce, look for a low•sugar or sugar•free variety, or make your own by mixing ketchup or tomato sauce with a bit of lemon juice, horseradish, and hot sauce.

- Serve the shrimp cocktail chilled for the best flavor and texture.

- Provide small cocktail forks or toothpicks to make it easy for guests to pick up the shrimp.

Shrimp cocktail is a classic appetizer that is perfect for those following a gastric bypass diet. The shrimp provides a lean source of protein, while the cocktail sauce adds a flavorful dipping option without too many added sugars or carbs.

This simple yet elegant dish makes a great starter or light snack. Adjust the portion size as needed to fit your dietary needs and enjoy this delicious shrimp cocktail!

62. Deviled eggs

Ingredients:

- 6 hard•boiled eggs
- 2 tbsp mayonnaise
- 1 tsp Dijon mustard
- 1 tsp white vinegar
- 1/4 tsp paprika
- Salt and pepper to taste
- Chopped chives or parsley for garnish (optional)

Instructions:

1. Peel the hard•boiled eggs and cut them in half lengthwise.

2. Carefully scoop the yolks out of the egg whites and place them in a small bowl.

3. Add the mayonnaise, Dijon mustard, white vinegar, paprika, and a pinch of salt and pepper to the bowl with the yolks. Mash and mix everything together until smooth and creamy.

4. Using a spoon or a piping bag, fill the egg white halves with the yolk mixture, dividing it evenly among the 12 egg halves.

5. Sprinkle the deviled eggs with a light dusting of paprika and garnish with chopped chives or parsley, if desired.

6. Refrigerate the deviled eggs until ready to serve.

Tips:
- Use full•fat or low•fat mayonnaise, depending on your dietary preferences.
- For a creamier texture, you can add a small amount of heavy cream or Greek yogurt to the yolk mixture.
- Experiment with different seasonings, such as cayenne pepper, garlic powder, or dill.
- Make ahead and refrigerate for up to 3 days.

Deviled eggs are a classic, protein•rich snack or appetizer that is perfect for those following a gastric bypass diet. The combination of hard•boiled eggs and a creamy, flavorful yolk filling makes for a satisfying and nutritious treat.

Adjust the portion size as needed to fit your dietary needs. Enjoy these delicious deviled eggs!

63. Smoked salmon rolls

Ingredients:

- 4 oz smoked salmon, thinly sliced
- 1/2 cup full•fat cream cheese, softened
- 2 tbsp chopped fresh dill
- 1 tbsp lemon juice
- 1/4 tsp black pepper
- 4 large lettuce leaves (such as romaine or butter lettuce)

Instructions:

1. In a small bowl, mix together the cream cheese, dill, lemon juice, and black pepper until well combined.

2. Lay a lettuce leaf flat on a clean surface. Spread about 2•3 tablespoons of the cream cheese mixture onto the center of the leaf.

3. Top the cream cheese with a few slices of smoked salmon, arranging them in a line down the center of the leaf.

4. Carefully roll up the lettuce leaf around the salmon and cream cheese, tucking in the sides as you go.

5. Repeat with the remaining lettuce leaves and filling to make 4 salmon rolls total.

6. Serve the smoked salmon rolls immediately, or refrigerate until ready to serve.

Optional Variations:
- Add a thin slice of cucumber or avocado to the rolls.
- Sprinkle the rolls with a pinch of everything bagel seasoning.
- Serve the rolls with a side of lemon wedges or a dollop of capers.

These smoked salmon rolls make a delicious and nutritious snack or light meal for those following a gastric bypass diet. The combination of healthy fats from the salmon and protein from the cream cheese provides a satisfying and filling option.

Adjust the portion size as needed to fit your dietary needs. Enjoy these fresh and flavorful smoked salmon rolls!

64. Chicken skewers with peanut sauce

Ingredients:

For the Chicken Skewers:
- 1 lb boneless, skinless chicken breasts, cut into 1•inch cubes
- 1 tbsp olive oil
- 1 tsp ground cumin
- 1 tsp garlic powder
- 1/2 tsp salt
- 1/4 tsp black pepper

For the Peanut Sauce:
- 1/2 cup creamy peanut butter
- 1/4 cup low•sodium soy sauce
- 2 tbsp rice vinegar
- 2 tbsp honey
- 1 tbsp freshly grated ginger
- 1 garlic clove, minced
- 1/4 tsp red pepper flakes (optional)
- 1/4 cup warm water

Instructions:

1. In a medium bowl, toss the chicken cubes with the olive oil, cumin, garlic powder, salt, and pepper until evenly coated.

2. Thread the chicken onto metal or wooden skewers, leaving a little space between each piece.

3. Preheat grill or grill pan to medium•high heat. Grill the chicken skewers for 2•3 minutes per side, or until cooked through.

4. In a small bowl, whisk together the peanut butter, soy sauce, rice vinegar, honey, ginger, garlic, and red pepper flakes (if using). Gradually whisk in the warm water until the sauce is smooth and creamy.

5. Serve the grilled chicken skewers warm, with the peanut sauce on the side for dipping.

Tips:
- Soak wooden skewers in water for 30 minutes before using to prevent burning.
- Adjust the amount of red pepper flakes to control the spice level.
- Serve the skewers with steamed rice, roasted vegetables, or a fresh salad.
- The peanut sauce can also be used as a marinade or dressing.

65. Mini meatballs

Ingredients:

- 1 lb ground beef (or a mix of ground beef and ground pork)
- 1 egg
- 1/2 cup breadcrumbs
- 1/4 cup grated Parmesan cheese
- 2 cloves garlic, minced
- 1 tsp dried oregano
- 1 tsp dried basil
- 1/2 tsp salt
- 1/4 tsp black pepper

Instructions:

1. Preheat your oven to 400°F (200°C). Line a baking sheet with parchment paper or a silicone baking mat.

2. In a large bowl, combine the ground beef, egg, breadcrumbs, Parmesan, garlic, oregano, basil, salt, and pepper. Mix well until all the ingredients are evenly distributed.

3. Using a small cookie scoop or spoon, form the mixture into 1•inch meatballs and place them on the prepared baking sheet, spacing them about 1 inch apart.

4. Bake the meatballs for 12•15 minutes, or until they are cooked through and lightly browned on the outside.

5. Serve the mini meatballs warm, either on their own as an appetizer or as a topping for pasta, salads, or sandwiches.

Tips:
- For extra flavor, you can add finely chopped onion, parsley, or other herbs to the meatball mixture.
- Use a combination of ground beef and ground pork for a more tender and flavorful meatball.
- If the meatball mixture is too wet, add a few more breadcrumbs. If it's too dry, add a bit of milk or water.
- Bake the meatballs in batches if needed, to ensure they cook evenly.
- Serve the meatballs with your favorite dipping sauce, such as marinara, pesto, or barbecue sauce.

These mini meatballs are perfect for parties, appetizers, or as a quick and easy addition to a variety of dishes. Enjoy!

66. Stuffed mushrooms with lean sausage

Ingredients:
- 12 large mushrooms, stems removed and finely chopped
- 1/2 lb lean Italian turkey or chicken sausage, casings removed
- 2 tbsp grated Parmesan cheese
- 2 tbsp cream cheese, softened
- 1 clove garlic, minced
- 1 tsp dried parsley
- 1/4 tsp black pepper

Instructions:
1. Preheat your oven to 375°F (190°C). Lightly grease a baking sheet or oven•safe dish.

2. Remove the stems from the mushrooms and finely chop them. Set the mushroom caps aside.

3. In a skillet over medium heat, cook the sausage, breaking it up with a wooden spoon, until browned and cooked through, about 5•7 minutes.

4. Add the chopped mushroom stems, garlic, parsley, and black pepper to the skillet. Sauté for an additional 2•3 minutes.

5. Remove the skillet from heat and stir in the Parmesan and cream cheese until well combined.

6. Spoon the sausage•cheese mixture into the mushroom caps, dividing it evenly.

7. Arrange the stuffed mushrooms on the prepared baking sheet or dish.

8. Bake for 12•15 minutes, or until the mushrooms are tender and the filling is hot and bubbly.

9. Serve the stuffed mushrooms warm.

Optional Variations:
- Top the stuffed mushrooms with a sprinkle of additional Parmesan or shredded mozzarella cheese.
- Add a pinch of red pepper flakes for a bit of heat.
- Substitute the sausage with ground turkey or chicken for an even leaner option.

These stuffed mushrooms are a delicious and protein•packed appetizer or snack that is perfect for those following a gastric bypass diet. The combination of lean sausage, cheese, and mushrooms provides a satisfying and flavorful bite.

67. Tuna tartare

Ingredients:

- 8 oz sushi•grade tuna, finely diced
- 1 tbsp sesame oil
- 1 tbsp soy sauce
- 1 tbsp rice vinegar
- 1 tsp sesame seeds
- 1 tsp finely chopped chives or green onions
- 1 tsp finely chopped cilantro (optional)
- 1/2 tsp grated ginger
- 1/4 tsp crushed red pepper flakes (optional)
- Salt and black pepper to taste

Serving Suggestions:

- Wonton crisps or crackers
- Avocado slices
- Cucumber slices
- Radish slices

Instructions:

1. In a medium bowl, gently mix together the diced tuna, sesame oil, soy sauce, rice vinegar, sesame seeds, chives/green onions, cilantro (if using), grated ginger, and red pepper flakes (if using). Season with salt and black pepper to taste.

2. Cover and refrigerate the tuna tartare for at least 30 minutes to allow the flavors to meld.

3. To serve, spoon the tuna tartare onto wonton crisps, crackers, or small plates. Garnish with sliced avocado, cucumber, or radish, if desired.

Tips:
- Use the freshest, sushi•grade tuna you can find for the best flavor and texture.
- Dice the tuna into very small, even cubes for the best presentation.
- Adjust the amounts of soy sauce, vinegar, and seasonings to your taste preferences.
- Serve the tuna tartare immediately after chilling to maintain its fresh, raw texture.
- For a heartier meal, serve the tuna tartare on top of a bed of mixed greens or rice.

Tuna tartare is a delicious and elegant appetizer or light main course. The combination of fresh tuna, Asian•inspired flavors, and crunchy garnishes makes for a truly delightful dish.

68. Eggplant chips with tzatziki

Ingredients:

- 1 large eggplant, sliced into 1/4•inch thick rounds
- 2 tbsp olive oil
- 1 tsp salt
- 1/2 tsp black pepper

Instructions:

1. Preheat oven to 400°F. Line 2 baking sheets with parchment paper.

2. Arrange the eggplant slices in a single layer on the prepared baking sheets. Brush the tops with olive oil and season with salt and pepper.

3. Bake for 15•20 minutes, flipping halfway, until the eggplant is golden brown and crispy.

4. Remove from oven and let cool completely before serving.

Tzatziki Sauce:
Ingredients:
- 1 cup plain Greek yogurt
- 1 cucumber, peeled, seeded and grated
- 1 garlic clove, minced
- 1 tbsp fresh lemon juice
- 1 tbsp chopped fresh dill
- 1/4 tsp salt
- 1/4 tsp black pepper

Instructions:
1. In a medium bowl, combine all the tzatziki ingredients and stir well to combine
.
2. Refrigerate for at least 30 minutes to allow the flavors to meld.

Serve the eggplant chips warm or at room temperature with the tzatziki sauce on the side for dipping. Enjoy!

69. Edamame with sea salt

Ingredients:

- 1 lb fresh edamame in the pod
- 2 tsp coarse sea salt

Instructions:

1. Bring a large pot of salted water to a boil. Add the edamame pods and cook for 5•7 minutes, until bright green and tender.

2. Drain the edamame and transfer to a serving bowl.

3. Sprinkle the coarse sea salt over the hot edamame and toss to coat evenly.

4. Serve the edamame warm, with the pods intact. Provide small dishes or bowls for guests to squeeze the edamame beans out of the pods and into their mouths.

Tips:

- Look for fresh, bright green edamame pods. Avoid any that are yellowed or dried out.

- The sea salt adds a nice crunch and salty flavor to the edamame.

- You can also try other seasonings like garlic powder, chili powder, or lemon zest.

- Edamame makes a great healthy snack or appetizer. The fiber and protein will help fill you up.

Enjoy your simple but tasty edamame with sea salt!

70. Cucumber and hummus bites

Ingredients:

- 1 large cucumber, sliced into 1/2•inch thick rounds
- 1 cup hummus (store•bought or homemade)
- 2 tbsp chopped fresh parsley or dill (optional)
- Paprika or za'atar seasoning (optional)

Instructions:

1. Slice the cucumber into 1/2•inch thick rounds. Pat the cucumber slices dry with a paper towel.

2. Spread about 1•2 tablespoons of hummus onto each cucumber slice, using the back of a spoon to smooth it out.

3. If desired, sprinkle the hummus•topped cucumber slices with a pinch of paprika, za'atar seasoning, or chopped fresh parsley or dill.

4. Arrange the cucumber and hummus bites on a serving platter or plate.

5. Refrigerate for at least 30 minutes before serving to allow the flavors to meld.

Tips:
- Use your favorite store•bought or homemade hummus flavor, such as classic, roasted red pepper, or garlic.
- For a creamier texture, you can mix a bit of Greek yogurt into the hummus.
- Try topping the bites with crumbled feta, chopped olives, or toasted pine nuts.
- These cucumber bites make a great healthy appetizer or snack. They're refreshing, flavorful, and easy to assemble.

Enjoy your cucumber and hummus bites!

71. Berry protein smoothie

Ingredients:

- 1 cup unsweetened almond milk
- 1/2 cup frozen mixed berries (such as blueberries, raspberries, and blackberries)
- 1 scoop (about 1/4 cup) vanilla or unflavored protein powder
- 1 tbsp ground flaxseed
- 1 tsp honey (optional)
- 1/2 cup ice cubes

Instructions:

1. Add all the ingredients to a high•powered blender.

2. Blend on high speed until the mixture is smooth and creamy, about 1 minute.

3. Pour the berry protein smoothie into a glass and enjoy immediately.

Optional Variations:
- Use fresh berries instead of frozen, if desired.

- Add a handful of spinach or kale for extra nutrients.

- Substitute the honey with a low•calorie sweetener like stevia or erythritol.

- Use a different protein powder flavor, such as chocolate or peanut butter.

- Top with a sprinkle of cinnamon or a few sliced almonds.

This berry protein smoothie is a great option for those following a gastric bypass diet. The combination of protein•rich powder, fiber•filled berries, and healthy fats from the flaxseed and almond milk makes it a nutritious and satisfying drink.

The smoothie provides a good amount of protein to help support your dietary needs, while the berries and flaxseed add beneficial nutrients like antioxidants, vitamins, and omega•3s.

Adjust the portion size as needed and enjoy this delicious and healthy berry protein smoothie as a snack or part of a balanced meal.

72. Green smoothie with spinach and protein powder

Ingredients:

- 1 cup fresh spinach leaves
- 1 banana, frozen
- 1/2 cup unsweetened almond milk (or milk of your choice)
- 1 scoop vanilla or unflavored protein powder
- 1 tbsp chia seeds or ground flaxseeds (optional)
- 1 cup ice cubes

Instructions:

1. Add the spinach, frozen banana, almond milk, protein powder, and chia/flax seeds (if using) to a high•powered blender.

2. Blend on high speed until the mixture is smooth and creamy, about 1•2 minutes.

3. Add the ice cubes and blend again until the smoothie is thick and frosty.

4. Pour into a glass and enjoy immediately.

Tips:
- Use fresh or frozen spinach • both work well.

- Adjust the amount of liquid to reach your desired consistency.

- Add a handful of other greens like kale or swiss chard for extra nutrients.

- Use a plant•based or whey protein powder.

- Top with sliced fruit, nuts, or a sprinkle of cinnamon if desired.

This green smoothie is a nutritious and filling breakfast or snack, providing fiber, vitamins, minerals, and plant•based protein. Adjust the ingredients to suit your taste preferences.

73. Peanut butter and banana protein smoothie

Ingredients:

- 1 ripe banana, frozen
- 2 tbsp creamy peanut butter
- 1 scoop vanilla or chocolate protein powder
- 1 cup unsweetened almond milk (or milk of your choice)
- 1 tbsp chia seeds or ground flaxseeds (optional)
- 1 cup ice cubes

Instructions:

1. Add the frozen banana, peanut butter, protein powder, almond milk, and chia/flax seeds (if using) to a high•powered blender.

2. Blend on high speed until the mixture is smooth and creamy, about 1•2 minutes.

3. Add the ice cubes and blend again until the smoothie is thick and frosty.

4. Pour into a glass and enjoy immediately.

Tips:
• Use a ripe, frozen banana for a naturally sweet and creamy smoothie.

• Adjust the amount of liquid to reach your desired consistency.

• Use a plant•based or whey protein powder.

• For extra protein, add a spoonful of Greek yogurt.

• Top with a sprinkle of cinnamon, crushed peanuts, or a drizzle of honey if desired.

This peanut butter banana protein smoothie is a delicious and nutritious way to start your day or refuel after a workout. The combination of protein, healthy fats, and carbohydrates makes it a balanced and satisfying smoothie.

74. Chocolate protein shake

Ingredients:

- 1 cup unsweetened almond milk (or milk of your choice)
- 1 scoop chocolate protein powder
- 1 frozen banana
- 1 tbsp unsweetened cocoa powder
- 1 tsp vanilla extract
- 1/2 tsp cinnamon (optional)
- 1•2 ice cubes (optional)

Instructions:

1. Add all the ingredients to a high•powered blender.

2. Blend on high speed until the mixture is smooth and creamy, about 1•2 minutes.

3. Taste and adjust any ingredients to your preference, such as adding more protein powder for a thicker shake or more almond milk for a thinner consistency.

4. Pour the chocolate protein shake into a glass and enjoy immediately.

Tips:
- Use a high•quality chocolate protein powder for the best flavor.

- Frozen banana adds natural sweetness and a thick, creamy texture.

- Cocoa powder enhances the chocolate flavor.

- Cinnamon provides a subtle warmth and pairs well with chocolate.

- Add a spoonful of peanut butter or almond butter for extra protein and healthy fats.

- Top with a sprinkle of cocoa powder, shredded coconut, or a few dark chocolate chips.

This chocolate protein shake is a delicious and nutritious way to refuel after a workout or enjoy as a healthy snack. The combination of protein, healthy fats, and complex carbs will keep you feeling satisfied and energized.

75. Tropical protein smoothie with mango and pineapple

Ingredients:

- 1 cup frozen mango chunks
- 1 cup frozen pineapple chunks
- 1 cup unsweetened almond milk (or milk of your choice)
- 1 scoop vanilla protein powder
- 1 tbsp chia seeds or ground flaxseeds
- 1 tsp honey (optional)
- 1/2 cup ice cubes

Instructions:

1. Add all the ingredients to a high•powered blender. Blend on high speed until smooth and creamy, about 1•2 minutes.

2. Taste and adjust sweetness if needed, adding a bit more honey if desired.

3. Pour the smoothie into a glass and enjoy immediately.

Tips:
• Use fresh or frozen fruit for best texture and flavor.

• Adjust the amount of milk to reach your desired consistency.

• Add a handful of spinach or kale for extra nutrients.

• Top with shredded coconut, sliced almonds, or a sprinkle of cinnamon.

This tropical smoothie is packed with protein, fiber, vitamins, and antioxidants from the mango, pineapple, and other ingredients. It makes a delicious and nutritious breakfast or snack.

76. Avocado and spinach smoothie

Ingredients:

- 1 ripe avocado, pitted and peeled
- 1 cup fresh spinach leaves
- 1 cup unsweetened almond milk (or milk of your choice)
- 1 banana, frozen
- 1 tbsp honey (optional)
- 1 tsp vanilla extract
- 1/2 cup ice cubes

Instructions:

1. Add all the ingredients to a high•powered blender. Blend on high speed until the mixture is smooth and creamy, about 1•2 minutes.

2. Taste and adjust sweetness by adding more honey if desired.

3. Pour the smoothie into glasses and serve immediately.

Tips:
- Use a ripe, soft avocado for the creamiest texture.

- Frozen banana adds natural sweetness and a thick, creamy consistency.

- Spinach provides a boost of nutrients without overpowering the flavor.

- Almond milk keeps the smoothie dairy•free, but you can use regular milk or another non•dairy milk.

- For extra protein, add a scoop of vanilla protein powder.

- Top with sliced avocado, a sprinkle of chia seeds, or a drizzle of nut butter.

This avocado and spinach smoothie is a nutritious and delicious way to start your day or enjoy as a healthy snack. The avocado provides healthy fats, while the spinach and banana offer fiber, vitamins, and minerals.

77. Strawberry and kale smoothie

Ingredients:

- 1 cup fresh or frozen strawberries
- 1 cup fresh kale, stems removed
- 1 banana, frozen
- 1 cup unsweetened almond milk (or milk of your choice)
- 1 tbsp honey or maple syrup (optional)
- 1 tbsp chia seeds or ground flaxseeds (optional)
- 1 cup ice cubes

Instructions:

1. Add all the ingredients to a high•powered blender. Blend on high speed until smooth and creamy, about 1•2 minutes.

2. Taste and adjust sweetener as needed. The banana and strawberries should provide enough natural sweetness, but you can add a bit of honey or maple syrup if desired.

3. Pour into a glass and enjoy immediately. You can also pour it into a reusable smoothie cup with a straw for on•the•go.

The kale provides a boost of nutrients like vitamins A, C, and K, as well as fiber. The strawberries and banana add natural sweetness and creaminess. The chia or flax seeds provide extra fiber, protein, and healthy omega•3s. This smoothie is a great way to start your day or have as a healthy snack.

78. Coffee protein smoothie

Ingredients:

- 1 cup unsweetened almond milk (or milk of your choice)
- 1 scoop vanilla or chocolate protein powder
- 1 frozen banana
- 1 tbsp instant coffee powder or 1 shot of espresso
- 1 tbsp peanut butter (or nut butter of your choice)
- 1 tbsp cocoa powder (optional)
- 1 tsp honey or maple syrup (optional)
- 1 cup ice cubes

Instructions:

1. Add all the ingredients to a high•powered blender. Blend on high speed until smooth and creamy, about 1•2 minutes.

2. Taste and adjust sweetener as needed. The banana and peanut butter should provide enough natural sweetness, but you can add a bit of honey or maple syrup if desired.

3. Pour into a glass and enjoy immediately. You can also pour it into a reusable smoothie cup with a straw for on•the•go.

The coffee and protein powder provide an energizing boost, while the banana, peanut butter, and milk create a rich, creamy texture. The cocoa powder adds a touch of chocolate flavor. This smoothie is perfect for a quick breakfast or post•workout recovery drink.

You can also customize the recipe by using different types of protein powder, nut butters, or even adding a handful of spinach or kale for extra nutrients.

79. Vanilla almond protein shake

Ingredients:

- 1 cup unsweetened almond milk
- 1 scoop vanilla protein powder
- 1 tbsp almond butter
- 1 tsp vanilla extract
- 1/2 banana, frozen
- 1/4 cup ice cubes

Instructions:

1. Add all the ingredients to a high•powered blender. Blend on high speed until smooth and creamy, about 1•2 minutes.

2. Taste and adjust any ingredients to your preference. Add more almond milk for a thinner consistency or more ice for a thicker shake.

3. Pour the shake into a glass and enjoy immediately.

Tips:
- Use a high•quality vanilla protein powder for best flavor.
- Substitute the banana with 1/2 cup of frozen cauliflower for a lower•carb option.
- Add a handful of spinach or kale for extra nutrients.
- Top with to

80. Blueberry and flaxseed smoothie

Ingredients:

- 1 cup fresh or frozen blueberries
- 1 banana, frozen
- 1 cup unsweetened almond milk (or milk of your choice)
- 1 tbsp ground flaxseeds
- 1 tbsp honey or maple syrup (optional)
- 1 cup ice cubes

Instructions:

1. Add all the ingredients to a high•powered blender. Blend on high speed until smooth and creamy, about 1•2 minutes.

2. Taste and adjust sweetener as needed. The banana and blueberries should provide enough natural sweetness, but you can add a bit of honey or maple syrup if desired.

3. Pour into a glass and enjoy immediately. You can also pour it into a reusable smoothie cup with a straw for on•the•go.

The blueberries provide antioxidants and fiber, while the flaxseeds add a boost of omega•3 fatty acids, fiber, and protein. The banana creates a creamy texture and natural sweetness. This smoothie is a great way to start your day or have as a healthy snack.

You can also customize the recipe by adding other fruits, greens like spinach or kale, nut butters, or even a scoop of protein powder. The possibilities are endless for creating a nutritious and delicious smoothie.

81. Grilled chicken Caesar salad

Ingredients:

- 2 boneless, skinless chicken breasts
- 2 tbsp olive oil
- 1 tsp garlic powder
- 1 tsp dried oregano
- Salt and pepper to taste
- 6 cups chopped romaine lettuce
- 1/2 cup shredded Parmesan cheese
- 1/4 cup Caesar salad dressing
- 1 cup croutons
- Lemon wedges for serving (optional)

Instructions:

1. Preheat grill or grill pan to medium•high heat.

2. Rub the chicken breasts with olive oil and season with garlic powder, oregano, salt, and pepper.

3. Grill the chicken for 5•7 minutes per side, or until cooked through. Let rest for 5 minutes, then slice or chop the chicken.

4. In a large salad bowl, combine the chopped romaine lettuce, grilled chicken, Parmesan cheese, and Caesar dressing. Toss to coat evenly.

5. Top the salad with croutons and serve with lemon wedges, if desired.

Tips:
- Use a high•quality Caesar dressing or make your own homemade version.
- Add other toppings like grilled or roasted vegetables, hard•boiled eggs, or bacon bits.
- For a heartier meal, serve the salad with a side of crusty bread or garlic bread.
- Marinate the chicken in the seasoning mixture for 30 minutes before grilling for extra flavor.

Enjoy this delicious and satisfying Grilled Chicken Caesar Salad!

82. Tuna salad with mixed greens

Ingredients:

- 2 (5 oz) cans of tuna, drained and flaked
- 2 tbsp mayonnaise
- 1 tbsp Dijon mustard
- 1 tbsp lemon juice
- 2 tbsp finely chopped celery
- 2 tbsp finely chopped red onion
- 2 tbsp chopped dill pickles (optional)
- Salt and pepper to taste
- 4 cups mixed greens (such as spinach, arugula, kale)
- 1 tomato, sliced
- 1/4 cup sliced cucumber
- 2 tbsp crumbled feta cheese (optional)

Instructions:

1. In a medium bowl, mix together the tuna, mayonnaise, Dijon mustard, lemon juice, celery, red onion, and pickles (if using). Season with salt and pepper to taste.

2. In a large salad bowl, arrange the mixed greens. Top with the tuna salad, sliced tomato, cucumber, and feta cheese (if using).

3. Serve immediately. You can also refrigerate the tuna salad separately and assemble the salad just before serving.

The tuna salad provides a good source of protein, while the mixed greens, tomato, and cucumber add fresh crunch and nutrients. The feta cheese adds a tangy, creamy element. This salad is a great option for a light, healthy lunch or dinner.

You can customize the tuna salad by adding other mix•ins like hard•boiled eggs, diced avocado, or chopped nuts. Serve it on a bed of lettuce or stuff it into a tomato or avocado half for a different presentation.

83. Quinoa and chickpea salad

Ingredients:

- 1 cup cooked quinoa, cooled
- 1 (15 oz) can chickpeas, drained and rinsed
- 1 cup diced cucumber
- 1 cup cherry tomatoes, halved
- 1/2 cup diced red onion
- 1/4 cup chopped fresh parsley
- 2 tbsp chopped fresh mint (optional)
- 2 tbsp olive oil
- 2 tbsp lemon juice
- 1 tsp Dijon mustard
- Salt and pepper to taste

Instructions:

1. In a large bowl, combine the cooked quinoa, chickpeas, cucumber, cherry tomatoes, red onion, parsley, and mint (if using).

2. In a small bowl, whisk together the olive oil, lemon juice, and Dijon mustard. Season with salt and pepper to taste.

3. Pour the dressing over the quinoa and chickpea mixture and toss gently to coat everything evenly.

4. Refrigerate the salad for at least 30 minutes to allow the flavors to meld. Serve chilled or at room temperature.

This salad is packed with protein from the quinoa and chickpeas, as well as fiber, vitamins, and minerals from the fresh vegetables. The lemon dressing adds a bright, tangy flavor that complements the other ingredients.

You can customize this salad by adding other vegetables like bell peppers, carrots, or zucchini. You can also swap out the herbs or use a different type of vinegar or citrus juice in the dressing. This salad is a great option for a healthy, filling lunch or side dish.

84. Shrimp and avocado salad

Ingredients:

- 1 lb cooked shrimp, peeled and deveined
- 2 avocados, diced
- 1 cup cherry tomatoes, halved
- 1/2 cup diced red onion
- 1/4 cup chopped fresh cilantro
- 2 tbsp olive oil
- 2 tbsp lime juice
- 1 tsp Dijon mustard
- Salt and pepper to taste

Instructions:

1. In a large bowl, combine the cooked shrimp, diced avocado, cherry tomatoes, red onion, and chopped cilantro.

2. In a small bowl, whisk together the olive oil, lime juice, and Dijon mustard. Season with salt and pepper to taste.

3. Pour the dressing over the shrimp and avocado mixture and toss gently to coat everything evenly.

4. Refrigerate the salad for at least 30 minutes to allow the flavors to meld. Serve chilled.

This salad is a delicious and healthy combination of protein•rich shrimp, creamy avocado, fresh vegetables, and a tangy lime dressing. The avocado provides healthy fats, while the shrimp adds lean protein. The cherry tomatoes and red onion add color, crunch, and flavor.

You can serve this salad on a bed of mixed greens or lettuce for a more substantial meal. It's also great as a standalone appetizer or side dish.

To customize the recipe, you can add other ingredients like diced cucumber, chopped mango, or crumbled feta cheese. You can also adjust the dressing to your taste, using different types of vinegar or adding a touch of honey or garlic.

85. Turkey and cranberry salad

Ingredients:

- 2 cups cooked and diced turkey breast
- 1/2 cup fresh or dried cranberries
- 2 tbsp chopped walnuts or pecans
- 2 tbsp plain Greek yogurt
- 1 tbsp Dijon mustard
- 1 tbsp lemon juice
- 1/4 tsp salt
- 1/4 tsp black pepper
- Mixed greens or lettuce leaves for serving

Instructions:

1. In a medium bowl, combine the diced turkey, cranberries, and chopped nuts.

2. In a small bowl, whisk together the Greek yogurt, Dijon mustard, lemon juice, salt, and pepper.

3. Pour the yogurt dressing over the turkey mixture and gently toss to coat.

4. Serve the turkey and cranberry salad on a bed of mixed greens or lettuce leaves.

Optional Variations:
- Add diced celery or apple for extra crunch.
- Substitute the walnuts or pecans with sliced almonds or chopped pistachios.
- Use a flavored Greek yogurt, such as honey or vanilla, for the dressing.
- Sprinkle the salad with a pinch of dried thyme or rosemary.

This turkey and cranberry salad is a delicious and nutritious option for those following a gastric bypass diet. The lean turkey provides a good source of protein, while the cranberries and nuts add fiber, healthy fats, and antioxidants.

The Greek yogurt•based dressing helps to keep the salad light and creamy without adding too many calories or carbs.

Adjust the portion size as needed to fit your dietary needs. Enjoy this flavorful and satisfying turkey and cranberry salad!

86. Greek salad with grilled chicken

Ingredients:

For the Salad:
• 6 cups chopped romaine lettuce
• 1 cup cherry tomatoes, halved
• 1 cucumber, diced
• 1/2 red onion, thinly sliced
• 1 cup crumbled feta cheese
• 1/2 cup Kalamata olives, pitted and halved
• 2 boneless, skinless chicken breasts

For the Dressing:
• 3 tbsp olive oil
• 2 tbsp red wine vinegar
• 1 tbsp lemon juice
• 1 tsp dried oregano
• 1 tsp Dijon mustard
• 1 garlic clove, minced
• Salt and pepper to taste

Instructions:

1. Preheat your grill or grill pan to medium•high heat. Season the chicken breasts with salt and pepper.

2. Grill the chicken for 5•7 minutes per side, or until cooked through. Allow the chicken to rest for 5 minutes, then slice or chop it.

3. In a large salad bowl, combine the chopped romaine lettuce, cherry tomatoes, diced cucumber, sliced red onion, crumbled feta cheese, and Kalamata olives.

4. In a small bowl, whisk together the olive oil, red wine vinegar, lemon juice, dried oregano, Dijon mustard, and minced garlic. Season with salt and pepper to taste.

5. Add the grilled chicken to the salad and drizzle the dressing over the top. Toss gently to coat everything evenly. Serve the Greek salad with grilled chicken immediately.

This Greek salad is a delicious and nutritious meal, with the grilled chicken providing a good source of protein. The fresh vegetables, tangy feta cheese, and briny olives create a flavorful and satisfying salad. The homemade Greek•inspired dressing ties all the flavors together

87. Spinach salad with boiled eggs

Ingredients:

- 6 cups fresh spinach leaves, washed and dried
- 4 hard•boiled eggs, peeled and sliced
- 1/2 cup sliced mushrooms
- 1/4 cup sliced red onion
- 2 tbsp crumbled feta cheese
- 2 tbsp toasted sunflower seeds or sliced almonds

For the Dressing:

- 2 tbsp olive oil
- 1 tbsp balsamic vinegar
- 1 tsp Dijon mustard
- 1 tsp honey
- Salt and pepper to taste

Instructions:

1. In a large salad bowl, combine the fresh spinach leaves, sliced hard•boiled eggs, mushrooms, red onion, feta cheese, and toasted sunflower seeds or almonds.

2. In a small bowl, whisk together the olive oil, balsamic vinegar, Dijon mustard, and honey. Season with salt and pepper to taste.

3. Drizzle the dressing over the spinach salad and toss gently to coat everything evenly.

4. Serve the spinach salad with boiled eggs immediately.

This spinach salad is a nutritious and filling meal, with the hard•boiled eggs providing a good source of protein. The mushrooms, red onion, and feta cheese add flavor and texture, while the toasted nuts or seeds provide a nice crunch.

The homemade balsamic vinaigrette dressing complements the fresh spinach and other ingredients perfectly.

You can customize this salad by adding other toppings like cherry tomatoes, avocado, or crispy bacon. It's a great option for a light lunch or a side dish for dinner.

Remember to adjust the quantities of the ingredients based on your personal preferences and the number of servings you need.

88. Caprese salad with added grilled chicken

Ingredients:

- 2 boneless, skinless chicken breasts
- 1 tbsp olive oil
- Salt and pepper to taste
- 8 oz fresh mozzarella cheese, sliced
- 2 cups cherry tomatoes, halved
- 1 cup fresh basil leaves
- 2 tbsp balsamic glaze
- 1 tbsp olive oil
- Salt and pepper to taste

Instructions:

1. Preheat your grill or grill pan to medium•high heat. Brush the chicken breasts with 1 tbsp of olive oil and season with salt and pepper.

2. Grill the chicken for 5•7 minutes per side, or until cooked through. Allow the chicken to rest for 5 minutes, then slice or shred it.

3. In a large serving bowl, arrange the sliced mozzarella, halved cherry tomatoes, and fresh basil leaves.

4. Top the Caprese salad with the grilled chicken.

5. Drizzle the balsamic glaze and remaining 1 tbsp of olive oil over the top. Season with additional salt and pepper to taste.

6. Serve immediately or refrigerate until ready to serve.

The combination of the fresh, creamy mozzarella, juicy tomatoes, and fragrant basil paired with the grilled chicken makes this Caprese salad a complete and satisfying meal. The balsamic glaze adds a sweet and tangy finish to the dish.

You can customize this recipe by using different types of tomatoes, such as heirloom or grape tomatoes. You can also add other ingredients like sliced avocado, roasted red peppers, or toasted pine nuts for extra flavor and texture.

This Caprese salad with grilled chicken is a great option for a light and healthy lunch or dinner, especially during the warmer months.

89. Black bean and corn salad with lean beef

Ingredients:

- 1 lb lean ground beef or ground turkey
- 1 (15 oz) can black beans, drained and rinsed
- 1 (15 oz) can corn, drained
- 1 cup diced tomatoes
- 1/2 cup diced red onion
- 1/4 cup chopped fresh cilantro
- 2 tbsp lime juice
- 1 tbsp olive oil
- 1 tsp chili powder
- 1/2 tsp cumin
- Salt and pepper to taste

Instructions:

1. In a large skillet, cook the ground beef or turkey over medium•high heat, breaking it up with a wooden spoon, until browned and cooked through, about 5•7 minutes. Drain any excess fat.

2. In a large bowl, combine the cooked ground beef, black beans, corn, diced tomatoes, red onion, and chopped cilantro.

3. In a small bowl, whisk together the lime juice, olive oil, chili powder, and cumin. Season with salt and pepper to taste.

4. Pour the dressing over the black bean and corn salad and toss gently to coat everything evenly.

5. Refrigerate the salad for at least 30 minutes to allow the flavors to meld.

6. Serve chilled or at room temperature.

This black bean and corn salad is a delicious and nutritious meal, with the lean ground beef or turkey providing a good source of protein. The black beans, corn, and fresh vegetables add fiber, vitamins, and minerals. The zesty lime dressing with chili powder and cumin complements the other ingredients perfectly.

You can customize this recipe by adding other ingredients like diced avocado, shredded cheese, or crushed tortilla chips. It's a great option for a light and healthy lunch or a side dish for dinner.

Remember to adjust the quantities of the ingredients based on your personal preferences and the number of servings you need.

90. Asian chicken salad with sesame dressing

Ingredients:

For the Salad:
• 2 cups shredded cooked chicken
• 4 cups mixed greens (such as romaine, cabbage, carrots)
• 1 cup shredded red cabbage
• 1 cup shredded purple cabbage
• 1/2 cup sliced cucumber
• 1/4 cup sliced green onions
• 2 tbsp toasted sesame seeds

For the Dressing:
• 2 tbsp sesame oil
• 2 tbsp rice vinegar
• 1 tbsp soy sauce
• 1 tbsp honey
• 1 tsp Dijon mustard
• 1 tsp grated ginger
• Salt and pepper to taste

Instructions:

1. In a large salad bowl, combine the shredded chicken, mixed greens, red and purple cabbage, cucumber, and green onions.

2. In a small bowl, whisk together all the dressing ingredients • sesame oil, rice vinegar, soy sauce, honey, Dijon mustard, and grated ginger. Season with salt and pepper to taste.

3. Pour the dressing over the salad and toss gently to coat everything evenly.

4. Sprinkle the toasted sesame seeds over the top of the salad.

5. Serve immediately or refrigerate until ready to serve.

The combination of tender chicken, crunchy vegetables, and the nutty sesame dressing makes this salad a delicious and nutritious meal. The Asian•inspired flavors from the soy sauce, ginger, and sesame oil complement the fresh ingredients perfectly.

You can customize this salad by adding other toppings like mandarin oranges, sliced almonds, crispy wonton strips, or shredded carrots. It's a great way to enjoy a healthy and satisfying lunch or dinner.

91. Baked chicken Parmesan with zucchini noodles

Ingredients:

For the Chicken Parmesan:
- 4 boneless, skinless chicken breasts
- 1 cup panko breadcrumbs
- 1/2 cup grated Parmesan cheese
- 1 tsp dried oregano
- 1/2 tsp garlic powder
- 1/4 tsp salt
- 1/4 tsp black pepper
- 1 egg, beaten
- 1 cup marinara sauce
- 1 cup shredded mozzarella cheese

For the Zucchini Noodles:
- 4 medium zucchini, spiralized or julienned
- 1 tbsp olive oil
- 1 garlic clove, minced
- Salt and pepper to taste

Instructions:

1. Preheat your oven to 400°F (200°C).

2. In a shallow bowl, combine the panko breadcrumbs, Parmesan cheese, oregano, garlic powder, salt, and pepper.

3. Dip the chicken breasts in the beaten egg, then coat them evenly with the breadcrumb mixture, pressing to adhere.

4. Place the breaded chicken on a baking sheet lined with parchment paper. Bake for 20•25 minutes, or until the chicken is cooked through and the breading is golden brown.

5. Top the baked chicken with the marinara sauce and shredded mozzarella cheese. Return to the oven and bake for an additional 5•10 minutes, or until the cheese is melted and bubbly.

6. While the chicken is baking, prepare the zucchini noodles. In a large skillet, heat the olive oil over medium heat. Add the minced garlic and sauté for 1 minute.

7. Add the spiralized or julienned zucchini noodles to the skillet and toss to coat with the garlic oil. Cook for 2•3 minutes, or until the zucchini noodles are tender but still have a bite.

8. Season the zucchini noodles with salt and pepper to taste.

9. Serve the baked chicken Parmesan on top of the zucchini noodle

92. Stuffed bell peppers with ground turkey

Ingredients:

- 4 large bell peppers (any color)
- 1 lb ground turkey
- 1 cup cooked brown rice
- 1 (15 oz) can diced tomatoes
- 1/2 cup diced onion
- 2 cloves garlic, minced
- 1 tsp dried oregano
- 1 tsp dried basil
- 1/2 tsp chili powder
- Salt and pepper to taste
- 1 cup shredded mozzarella cheese

Instructions:

1. Preheat your oven to 375°F (190°C).

2. Cut the tops off the bell peppers and remove the seeds and membranes. Place the peppers in a baking dish and set aside.

3. In a large skillet, cook the ground turkey over medium heat, breaking it up with a wooden spoon, until browned and cooked through, about 5•7 minutes. Drain any excess fat.

4. Add the cooked brown rice, diced tomatoes, onion, garlic, oregano, basil, chili powder, and salt and pepper to the skillet with the ground turkey. Stir to combine.

5. Spoon the turkey and rice mixture into the hollowed•out bell peppers, packing it in tightly.

6. Top each stuffed pepper with shredded mozzarella cheese.

7. Cover the baking dish with foil and bake for 30•35 minutes, or until the peppers are tender and the cheese is melted and bubbly.

8. Remove the foil during the last 5 minutes of baking to allow the cheese to brown slightly. Serve the stuffed bell peppers hot.

These stuffed bell peppers are a delicious and healthy meal, with the ground turkey providing lean protein and the bell peppers and rice adding fiber and nutrients. The melted mozzarella cheese on top adds a creamy, comforting touch.

93. Grilled steak with a side salad

Ingredients:

For the Steak:
- 2 (8 oz) ribeye or New York strip steaks
- 2 tbsp olive oil
- 2 tsp garlic powder
- 2 tsp onion powder
- 1 tsp dried thyme
- Salt and pepper to taste

For the Salad:
- 4 cups mixed greens (such as spinach, arugula, and romaine)
- 1 cup cherry tomatoes, halved
- 1/2 cup sliced cucumber
- 1/4 cup sliced red onion
- 2 tbsp crumbled feta cheese
- 2 tbsp balsamic vinaigrette

Instructions:

For the Steak:
1. Pat the steaks dry with paper towels and season both sides generously with the garlic powder, onion powder, dried thyme, salt, and pepper.
2. Heat a grill or grill pan to medium•high heat. Brush the steaks with the olive oil.
3. Grill the steaks for 4•6 minutes per side, or until they reach your desired level of doneness. Let the steaks rest for 5 minutes before slicing.

For the Salad:
1. In a large salad bowl, combine the mixed greens, cherry tomatoes, sliced cucumber, red onion, and crumbled feta cheese.
2. Drizzle the balsamic vinaigrette over the salad and toss gently to coat.

To Serve:
1. Slice the grilled steak and arrange it on a plate or platter.
2. Serve the side salad alongside the grilled steak.

This grilled steak with a side salad is a classic and nutritious meal. The juicy, flavorful steak provides a good source of protein, while the fresh salad adds fiber, vitamins, and minerals. The balsamic vinaigrette dressing complements the steak and salad perfectly.

You can customize this recipe by using different cuts of steak, adding more vegetables to the salad, or using a different type of dressing. Enjoy this delicious and well•balanced meal!

94. Pork chops with apple compote

Ingredients:

- 4 boneless pork chops (about 1 lb total)
- 1 tbsp olive oil
- 1 tsp dried thyme
- Salt and pepper to taste
- 2 apples, peeled, cored, and diced
- 1/4 cup unsweetened apple juice or cider
- 1 tbsp lemon juice
- 1/2 tsp ground cinnamon
- 1/4 tsp ground nutmeg

Instructions:

1. Preheat your oven to 400°F (200°C).

2. Season the pork chops on both sides with the dried thyme, salt, and pepper.

3. In a large oven•safe skillet or cast•iron pan, heat the olive oil over medium•high heat. Add the pork chops and sear for 2•3 minutes per side until browned.

4. Transfer the skillet to the preheated oven and bake the pork chops for 12•15 minutes, or until they reach an internal temperature of 145°F (63°C).

5. While the pork chops are baking, prepare the apple compote. In a small saucepan, combine the diced apples, apple juice or cider, lemon juice, cinnamon, and nutmeg.

6. Bring the apple mixture to a simmer over medium heat, stirring occasionally, until the apples are softened and the sauce has thickened, about 10•12 minutes.

7. Remove the pork chops from the oven and let them rest for 5 minutes.

8. Serve the pork chops warm, topped with the apple compote.

Optional Garnishes:
- Chopped fresh parsley or thyme
- A drizzle of balsamic glaze

This pork chops with apple compote dish is a delicious and nutritious option for those following a gastric bypass diet. The lean pork provides protein, while the apples and spices add natural sweetness and fiber.

95. Chicken fajitas with lettuce wraps

Ingredients:

- 1 lb boneless, skinless chicken breasts, sliced into thin strips
- 2 tbsp olive oil
- 1 tbsp fajita seasoning (or a mix of chili powder, cumin, garlic powder, and paprika)
- 1 red bell pepper, sliced
- 1 green bell pepper, sliced
- 1 onion, sliced
- 1 lime, juiced
- Salt and pepper to taste
- 12•16 large lettuce leaves (such as romaine or bibb lettuce)
- Optional toppings: guacamole, salsa, sour cream, shredded cheese

Instructions:

1. In a large skillet or wok, heat the olive oil over medium•high heat.

2. Add the sliced chicken and fajita seasoning. Cook, stirring occasionally, until the chicken is cooked through and lightly browned, about 6•8 minutes.

3. Add the sliced bell peppers and onion to the skillet. Continue to cook, stirring frequently, until the vegetables are tender•crisp, about 5•7 minutes.

4. Squeeze the lime juice over the chicken and vegetable mixture. Toss to combine.

5. Season with salt and pepper to taste.

6. To serve, place a few slices of the chicken and vegetable mixture into a lettuce leaf. Top with your desired toppings, such as guacamole, salsa, sour cream, or shredded cheese.

7. Repeat with the remaining lettuce leaves and filling.

These chicken fajitas with lettuce wraps are a healthy and low•carb alternative to traditional fajitas served in tortillas. The crisp lettuce leaves provide a refreshing and crunchy base for the flavorful chicken and vegetables.

You can customize the fillings by using different types of peppers, adding mushrooms or zucchini, or using a different protein like shrimp or tofu.

Serve the lettuce wrap fajitas with a side of black beans or a fresh salad for a complete and satisfying meal.

96. Baked swordfish with lemon and herbs

Ingredients:

- 4 (6 oz) swordfish steaks
- 2 tbsp olive oil
- 2 tbsp freshly squeezed lemon juice
- 2 tsp grated lemon zest
- 2 garlic cloves, minced
- 2 tbsp chopped fresh parsley
- 1 tbsp chopped fresh thyme
- 1 tsp dried oregano
- Salt and pepper to taste

Instructions:

1. Preheat your oven to 400°F (200°C).

2. In a small bowl, whisk together the olive oil, lemon juice, lemon zest, minced garlic, chopped parsley, chopped thyme, and dried oregano. Season with salt and pepper to taste.

3. Place the swordfish steaks in a baking dish or on a rimmed baking sheet. Pour the lemon•herb mixture over the swordfish, making sure to coat the fish evenly on both sides.

4. Bake the swordfish for 12•15 minutes, or until it flakes easily with a fork and is opaque throughout.

5. Serve the baked swordfish immediately, garnished with any remaining lemon•herb mixture from the baking dish.

This baked swordfish dish is a simple yet flavorful way to prepare this firm, meaty fish. The lemon and herb marinade adds a bright, fresh taste that complements the swordfish perfectly.

Swordfish is a great source of protein, as well as being rich in omega•3 fatty acids, vitamins, and minerals. Baking the fish helps to keep it moist and tender.

You can serve the baked swordfish with roasted vegetables, a fresh salad, or a side of quinoa or rice for a complete and healthy meal. Enjoy!

97. Tofu and vegetable stir•fry

Ingredients:

- 1 block (14 oz) extra•firm tofu, drained and cubed
- 2 tbsp sesame oil
- 2 cloves garlic, minced
- 1 inch piece fresh ginger, peeled and grated
- 1 red bell pepper, sliced
- 1 cup broccoli florets
- 1 cup sliced mushrooms
- 1 cup snow peas or snap peas
- 2 tbsp low•sodium soy sauce
- 1 tbsp rice vinegar
- 1 tsp honey
- Salt and pepper to taste
- Chopped green onions and sesame seeds for garnish (optional)

Instructions:

1. In a large skillet or wok, heat the sesame oil over medium•high heat.

2. Add the cubed tofu and cook, stirring occasionally, until lightly browned on all sides, about 5•7 minutes. Transfer the tofu to a plate and set aside.

3. In the same skillet, add the minced garlic and grated ginger. Cook for 1 minute, stirring constantly, until fragrant.

4. Add the sliced bell pepper, broccoli florets, mushrooms, and snow peas or snap peas. Stir•fry the vegetables for 3•5 minutes, or until they are tender•crisp.

5. Return the cooked tofu to the skillet. Add the soy sauce, rice vinegar, and honey. Toss everything together and cook for an additional 2•3 minutes, until the sauce has thickened slightly.

6. Season the stir•fry with salt and pepper to taste. Serve the tofu and vegetable stir•fry hot, garnished with chopped green onions and sesame seeds, if desired.

This tofu and vegetable stir•fry is a delicious and nutritious meatless meal. The firm tofu provides a good source of plant•based protein, while the colorful vegetables add fiber, vitamins, and minerals. The savory•sweet sauce ties all the flavors together.

You can customize this recipe by using different vegetables, such as bok choy, carrots, or zucchini. You can also adjust the sauce ingredients to your taste preferences.

98. Beef and vegetable kabobs

Ingredients:

- 1 lb beef sirloin or tenderloin, cut into 1•inch cubes
- 1 red bell pepper, cut into 1•inch pieces
- 1 yellow bell pepper, cut into 1•inch pieces
- 1 red onion, cut into 1•inch pieces
- 8 oz mushrooms, halved
- 1 zucchini, cut into 1•inch pieces
- 2 tbsp olive oil
- 2 tbsp balsamic vinegar
- 2 tsp dried oregano
- 1 tsp garlic powder
- Salt and pepper to taste
- Wooden or metal skewers

Instructions:

1. In a large bowl, combine the cubed beef, bell pepper pieces, onion pieces, mushrooms, and zucchini pieces.

2. In a small bowl, whisk together the olive oil, balsamic vinegar, dried oregano, and garlic powder. Season with salt and pepper to taste.

3. Pour the marinade over the beef and vegetables and toss to coat everything evenly. Cover and refrigerate for at least 30 minutes, or up to 2 hours.

4. Preheat your grill or grill pan to medium•high heat.

5. Thread the marinated beef and vegetables onto the skewers, alternating the ingredients.

6. Grill the kabobs for 10•12 minutes, turning occasionally, until the beef is cooked to your desired doneness and the vegetables are tender•crisp.

7. Serve the beef and vegetable kabobs hot, with any remaining marinade drizzled over the top.

These beef and vegetable kabobs are a delicious and healthy grilled meal. The combination of tender beef, crisp vegetables, and the flavorful balsamic marinade makes for a satisfying and nutritious dish.

You can customize the kabobs by using different types of meat (such as chicken or shrimp) or by swapping in your favorite vegetables (like mushrooms, cherry tomatoes, or pineapple chunks).

99. Grilled lamb chops with mint yogurt sauce

Ingredients:

For the Lamb Chops:
- 8 lamb chops (about 1•inch thick)
- 2 tbsp olive oil
- 2 tsp dried oregano
- 1 tsp garlic powder
- Salt and pepper to taste

For the Mint Yogurt Sauce:
- 1 cup plain Greek yogurt
- 2 tbsp chopped fresh mint
- 1 tbsp lemon juice
- 1 garlic clove, minced
- 1/4 tsp salt

Instructions:

1. In a shallow dish, combine the olive oil, oregano, garlic powder, salt, and pepper. Add the lamb chops and turn to coat them evenly with the seasoning mixture. Cover and let marinate for 30 minutes to 1 hour.

2. Preheat your grill or grill pan to medium•high heat.

3. Grill the lamb chops for 4•5 minutes per side, or until they reach the desired level of doneness. The internal temperature should reach 145°F (63°C) for medium•rare or 160°F (71°C) for medium.

4. While the lamb chops are grilling, prepare the mint yogurt sauce. In a small bowl, mix together the Greek yogurt, chopped mint, lemon juice, minced garlic, and salt.

5. Serve the grilled lamb chops warm, with the mint yogurt sauce spooned over the top or served on the side.

The combination of the juicy, flavorful lamb chops and the cool, refreshing mint yogurt sauce creates a delicious and balanced meal. The mint and lemon in the sauce complement the rich, savory lamb perfectly.

You can adjust the cooking time for the lamb chops based on your preferred level of doneness. Serve the grilled lamb chops with roasted vegetables, a fresh salad, or a side of couscous or rice for a complete and satisfying meal.

100. Stuffed portobello mushrooms with ricotta and spinach

Ingredients:

- 4 large portobello mushroom caps, stems removed and chopped
- 1 tbsp olive oil
- 1/2 cup diced onion
- 2 garlic cloves, minced
- 2 cups fresh spinach, chopped
- 1 cup part•skim ricotta cheese
- 1/4 cup grated Parmesan cheese
- 1 tsp dried oregano
- 1/4 tsp red pepper flakes (optional)
- Salt and pepper to taste
- 1/2 cup shredded mozzarella cheese

Instructions:

1. Preheat your oven to 400°F (200°C).

2. Gently clean the portobello mushroom caps with a damp paper towel. Remove and chop the stems.

3. In a skillet, heat the olive oil over medium heat. Add the chopped mushroom stems, diced onion, and minced garlic. Sauté for 3•4 minutes, until the onions are translucent.

4. Add the chopped spinach to the skillet and cook for an additional 2•3 minutes, until the spinach is wilted. Remove from heat and let cool slightly.

5. In a medium bowl, mix together the sautéed mushroom stem and spinach mixture, ricotta cheese, Parmesan cheese, dried oregano, and red pepper flakes (if using). Season with salt and pepper to taste.

6. Arrange the portobello mushroom caps, gill•side up, on a baking sheet or in a baking dish. Spoon the ricotta and spinach filling evenly into the mushroom caps.

7. Top each stuffed mushroom with a sprinkle of shredded mozzarella cheese. Bake for 15•20 minutes, or until the mushrooms are tender and the cheese is melted and bubbly. Serve the stuffed portobello mushrooms hot.

These stuffed portobello mushrooms make a delicious and healthy vegetarian main dish or appetizer. The combination of creamy ricotta, fresh spinach, and savory Parmesan cheese creates a flavorful filling that complements the meaty mushroom caps.

101. Protein•infused water

Ingredients:

- 1 gallon (4 liters) of water
- 1 scoop of unflavored whey protein powder or plant•based protein powder
- Sliced fruit or herbs (optional)

Instructions:

1. In a large pitcher or water dispenser, add the water and the protein powder. Whisk or stir vigorously until the protein powder is fully dissolved.

2. For added flavor and nutrients, you can also add sliced fruit like lemon, lime, orange, cucumber, or berries. Herbs like mint, basil, or rosemary also work well.

3. Refrigerate the protein•infused water for at least 2 hours to allow the flavors to infuse.

4. Serve chilled over ice. Refill the pitcher as needed, stirring or whisking the protein powder back into the water.

The benefits of protein•infused water include:

- Increased protein intake throughout the day to support muscle recovery and growth
- Hydration with added nutrients and antioxidants from the fruit or herbs
- A refreshing, lightly flavored alternative to plain water
- Convenience of having a protein•rich beverage on hand

You can experiment with different protein powders, fruit, and herb combinations to find your favorite flavor profile. Start with 1 scoop of protein powder per gallon of water and adjust to your taste preferences.

This protein•infused water is great for sipping throughout the day, before or after workouts, or as a healthy replacement for sugary drinks. Enjoy!

102. Green tea with added collagen

Ingredients:

- 1 cup hot water
- 1 green tea bag or 1 tsp loose leaf green tea
- 1 scoop (about 10•15 grams) of unflavored collagen powder

Instructions:

1. Bring 1 cup of water to a boil.

2. Place the green tea bag or loose leaf tea in a mug or teapot. Pour the hot water over the tea and let it steep for 3•5 minutes.

3. Remove the tea bag or strain out the loose leaf tea leaves.

4. Add the scoop of unflavored collagen powder to the brewed green tea and stir until it's fully dissolved.

5. Enjoy your green tea with collagen while it's hot.

The benefits of this green tea with collagen drink include:

- Antioxidants from the green tea to support overall health
- Collagen to help support skin, hair, nail, and joint health
- Hydration from the water
- No added sugars or artificial ingredients

You can customize this recipe in a few ways:

- Use matcha green tea powder instead of brewed green tea
- Add a squeeze of lemon or a drizzle of honey for extra flavor
- Blend the green tea and collagen with ice for an iced version
- Try different flavors of collagen powder, such as vanilla or chocolate

This green tea with collagen is a great way to incorporate more of this beneficial protein into your daily routine. Enjoy it as a healthy beverage any time of day.

Remember to consult your healthcare provider before adding any new supplements to your diet, especially if you have any underlying health conditions.

103. Protein hot chocolate

Ingredients:

- 1 cup unsweetened almond milk (or milk of your choice)
- 1 scoop chocolate or vanilla protein powder
- 1 tbsp unsweetened cocoa powder
- 1 tsp honey or maple syrup (optional)
- 1/4 tsp ground cinnamon (optional)
- Pinch of salt

Instructions:

1. In a small saucepan, whisk together the almond milk, protein powder, cocoa powder, honey/maple syrup (if using), cinnamon (if using), and a pinch of salt.

2. Heat the mixture over medium heat, whisking frequently, until it's hot and the ingredients are fully combined, about 3•5 minutes. Do not let it boil.

3. Remove the saucepan from the heat and pour the protein hot chocolate into a mug.

4. Optionally, you can top the hot chocolate with a dollop of whipped cream, a sprinkle of cocoa powder, or a cinnamon stick for garnish.

5. Serve the protein hot chocolate immediately while it's hot.

The benefits of this protein hot chocolate include:

- Protein from the protein powder to support muscle recovery and growth
- Antioxidants and flavor from the unsweetened cocoa powder
- Natural sweetness from the honey or maple syrup (optional)
- Warmth and coziness for a comforting treat

You can customize this recipe in a few ways:

- Use different types of protein powder, such as vanilla, mocha, or peanut butter
- Substitute the almond milk with another milk of your choice (dairy, oat, etc.)
- Add a splash of vanilla extract or a pinch of cayenne pepper for extra flavor
- Top with crushed nuts, shredded coconut, or a drizzle of melted dark chocolate

This protein hot chocolate is a delicious and nutritious way to satisfy your sweet tooth and get a protein boost. Enjoy it as a healthy treat on a cold day or as a post•workout recovery drink.

104. Almond milk latte with protein powder

Ingredients:

- 1 cup unsweetened almond milk
- 1 shot (1•2 oz) of espresso or strong brewed coffee
- 1 scoop of vanilla or chocolate protein powder
- 1 tsp honey or maple syrup (optional)
- Ground cinnamon for dusting (optional)

Instructions:

1. In a small saucepan, heat the almond milk over medium heat, stirring frequently, until it's steaming and frothy, about 2•3 minutes. Be careful not to let it boil.

2. In a mug, combine the hot espresso or coffee with the protein powder and stir until the powder is fully dissolved.

3. Carefully pour the steamed and frothed almond milk into the mug with the coffee•protein mixture. Stir gently to combine.

4. If desired, stir in 1 tsp of honey or maple syrup to sweeten the latte.

5. Top the latte with a light dusting of ground cinnamon.

6. Serve the almond milk latte with protein powder immediately while it's hot.

The benefits of this almond milk latte with protein powder include:

- Protein from the protein powder to support muscle recovery and growth
- Caffeine from the espresso or coffee for an energy boost
- Creaminess and natural sweetness from the almond milk and optional honey/maple syrup
- Antioxidants and flavor from the cinnamon

You can customize this recipe by using different types of protein powder, such as chocolate or mocha flavors. You can also experiment with other milk alternatives, like oat or soy milk.

This almond milk latte with protein powder is a delicious and nutritious way to start your day or enjoy as a mid•afternoon pick•me•up. Enjoy this creamy, energizing beverage!

105. Matcha protein shake

Ingredients:

- 1 cup unsweetened almond milk (or milk of your choice)
- 1 scoop vanilla or unflavored protein powder
- 1 tsp matcha green tea powder
- 1 frozen banana
- 1 tbsp almond butter (or nut butter of your choice)
- 1 tsp honey (optional)
- 1 cup ice cubes

Instructions:

1. Add all the ingredients to a high•powered blender. Blend on high speed until smooth and creamy, about 1•2 minutes.

2. Taste and adjust sweetener as needed. The banana and honey (if using) should provide enough natural sweetness, but you can add more honey to taste.

3. Pour the matcha protein shake into a glass and enjoy immediately.

The benefits of this matcha protein shake include:

- Protein from the protein powder to support muscle recovery and growth
- Antioxidants and a natural energy boost from the matcha green tea powder
- Healthy fats and fiber from the almond butter
- Natural sweetness and creaminess from the banana
- Hydration from the almond milk

You can customize this recipe by using different types of protein powder, nut butters, or even adding a handful of spinach or kale for extra nutrients.

This matcha protein shake is a great option for a post•workout recovery drink, a healthy breakfast, or an afternoon pick•me•up. The combination of protein, healthy fats, and antioxidants makes it a nutritious and satisfying beverage.

Enjoy this delicious and energizing matcha protein shake!

106. Herbal tea with a scoop of protein powder

Ingredients:

- 1 cup hot water
- 1 herbal tea bag (such as chamomile, peppermint, or ginger)
- 1 scoop unflavored or vanilla protein powder
- 1 tsp honey (optional)

Instructions:

1. Bring 1 cup of water to a boil.

2. Place the herbal tea bag in a mug and pour the hot water over it. Allow the tea to steep for 5•7 minutes.

3. Remove the tea bag and stir in the protein powder until it's fully dissolved.

4. If desired, stir in 1 tsp of honey to add a touch of sweetness.

5. Enjoy the warm, protein•infused herbal tea.

Tips:
• Use an unflavored or vanilla•flavored protein powder so it doesn't clash with the herbal tea flavor.

• Try different herbal tea varieties like chamomile for relaxation, peppermint for digestion, or ginger for immune support.

• Adjust the amount of protein powder to your preference, starting with 1 scoop.

• The honey is optional, but can help balance any bitterness from the protein powder.

• You can also add a squeeze of lemon or a sprinkle of cinnamon for extra flavor.

This protein•infused herbal tea makes a great post•workout recovery drink or a soothing bedtime beverage. The protein helps support muscle recovery and the herbs provide additional health benefits.

107. Low•sugar electrolyte drinks

Ingredients:

- 4 cups water
- 1/4 cup freshly squeezed lemon or lime juice
- 1/4 cup unsweetened coconut water
- 1 tablespoon honey or maple syrup (optional)
- 1/4 teaspoon sea salt
- 1/4 teaspoon potassium chloride (salt substitute)

Instructions:

1. In a large pitcher or container, combine the water, lemon/lime juice, coconut water, honey/maple syrup (if using), sea salt, and potassium chloride. Stir well until the salt and sweetener (if using) have dissolved.

2. Taste and adjust any ingredients as needed. You may want to add a bit more lemon/lime juice, sweetener, or salt depending on your taste preferences.

3. Chill the electrolyte drink in the refrigerator for at least 30 minutes before serving over ice.

4. Enjoy the drink chilled. It can be stored in the fridge for up to 5 days.

Notes:
- The coconut water provides natural electrolytes like potassium, while the lemon/lime juice provides vitamin C and electrolytes.
- The honey or maple syrup is optional if you want to add a touch of sweetness. You can also omit it for a completely unsweetened version.
- The potassium chloride helps replenish electrolytes lost through sweat.
- Feel free to experiment with different citrus juices or add fresh herbs like mint or basil.

This low•sugar electrolyte drink is perfect for rehydrating and replenishing after exercise, hot weather, or illness. It's a healthier alternative to commercial sports drinks.

108. Iced coffee with protein powder

Ingredients:

- 1 cup brewed coffee, chilled
- 1 scoop vanilla or chocolate protein powder
- 1 cup unsweetened almond milk (or milk of your choice)
- 1•2 tsp honey or maple syrup (optional)
- Ice cubes

Instructions:

1. In a blender, combine the chilled coffee, protein powder, and almond milk. Blend on high speed until smooth and frothy.

2. Taste the iced coffee and add 1•2 tsp of honey or maple syrup if you'd like it to be a bit sweeter.

3. Fill a glass with ice cubes.

4. Pour the blended iced coffee over the ice.

5. Serve immediately and enjoy!

The benefits of this iced coffee with protein powder include:

- Increased protein intake to support muscle recovery and growth
- Caffeine from the coffee for an energy boost
- Hydration from the almond milk
- Optional sweetener for a touch of natural sweetness

You can customize this recipe in a few ways:

- Use different types of protein powder, such as chocolate, mocha, or vanilla
- Substitute the almond milk with another milk of your choice (dairy, oat, etc.)
- Add a splash of vanilla extract or a pinch of cinnamon for extra flavor
- Blend in a frozen banana for a creamier, smoothie•like texture

This iced coffee with protein powder is a great option for a refreshing and nutritious pick•me•up, especially after a workout or as a mid•afternoon snack. Enjoy this delicious and energizing beverage!

109. Protein•infused green juice

Ingredients:

- 1 cup spinach
- 1 cup kale
- 1 cucumber, peeled and chopped
- 1 apple, cored and chopped
- 1 lemon, peeled
- 1 inch fresh ginger, peeled
- 1 scoop vanilla or unflavored protein powder
- 1/2 cup water or unsweetened almond milk

Instructions:

1. Add the spinach, kale, cucumber, apple, lemon, and ginger to a high•powered blender or juicer.

2. Blend or juice the ingredients until smooth and liquefied.

3. Add the protein powder and water/almond milk. Blend again until fully incorporated.

4. Pour the green juice into a glass and enjoy immediately.

Tips:
- Use a high•quality plant•based or whey protein powder for the best flavor and texture.
- Adjust the amount of water/milk to reach your desired consistency.
- You can also add other greens like parsley or celery for extra nutrients.
- For sweetness, add a touch of honey or maple syrup.

This protein•packed green juice is a great way to start your day or refuel after a workout. The combination of leafy greens, fruit, and protein powder provides a nutrient•dense boost of energy and antioxidants. Enjoy!

110. Berry•infused water with added protein

Ingredients:

- 4 cups water
- 1 cup mixed berries (such as raspberries, blueberries, strawberries)
- 1 scoop vanilla or unflavored protein powder
- 1 tbsp honey (optional)

Instructions:

1. In a large pitcher or water bottle, combine the water and mixed berries. Gently muddle the berries with a wooden spoon to release their juices.

2. Add the protein powder and stir or shake vigorously until the powder is fully dissolved.

3. If desired, stir in the honey to add a touch of sweetness.

4. Refrigerate the berry protein water for at least 2 hours, or up to 24 hours, to allow the flavors to infuse.

5. Serve the berry protein water over ice. You can also top it off with a few extra fresh berries.

Tips:
- Use a high•quality plant•based or whey protein powder for the best flavor and texture.

- Try different berry combinations like strawberry•kiwi or blackberry•lemon.

- Adjust the amount of protein powder to your preference, starting with 1 scoop.

- The honey is optional, but can help balance any bitterness from the protein powder.

- For a fizzy version, use sparkling water instead of still water.

This refreshing berry•infused protein water is a great way to stay hydrated and get an extra protein boost. It's perfect for sipping on a hot day or as a post•workout recovery drink. Enjoy!

111. Cottage cheese and fruit bowl

Ingredients:

- 1 cup low•fat or non•fat cottage cheese
- 1 cup mixed fresh fruit (such as berries, diced apple, diced mango, etc.)
- 1 tbsp honey or maple syrup (optional)
- 1 tbsp chopped nuts or seeds (such as almonds, walnuts, or chia seeds)

Instructions:

1. In a medium bowl, scoop out the cottage cheese and smooth it out with the back of a spoon.

2. Top the cottage cheese with the mixed fresh fruit. Arrange the fruit in a visually appealing way.

3. If desired, drizzle the honey or maple syrup over the fruit and cottage cheese.

4. Sprinkle the chopped nuts or seeds over the top.

5. Serve the cottage cheese and fruit bowl immediately, or refrigerate until ready to enjoy.

This cottage cheese and fruit bowl is a simple, yet nutritious and satisfying snack or light meal. The benefits include:

- Protein from the cottage cheese to help keep you feeling full and satisfied
- Vitamins, minerals, and fiber from the fresh fruit
- Healthy fats and crunch from the nuts or seeds
- Optional sweetness from the honey or maple syrup

You can customize this recipe by using your favorite fruits, such as berries, citrus, stone fruits, or tropical fruits. You can also experiment with different types of nuts, seeds, or even a sprinkle of granola.

This cottage cheese and fruit bowl is a great option for breakfast, a mid•afternoon snack, or a light dessert. It's a simple, yet nutritious and delicious way to enjoy a balance of protein, carbohydrates, and healthy fats.

Enjoy this refreshing and satisfying cottage cheese and fruit bowl!

112. Tofu with peanut sauce and vegetables

Ingredients:

- 1 block (14 oz) extra•firm tofu, cubed
- 2 tbsp sesame oil
- 1 cup broccoli florets
- 1 cup sliced carrots
- 1 red bell pepper, sliced
- 2 cloves garlic, minced
- 1/4 cup creamy peanut butter
- 2 tbsp low•sodium soy sauce
- 1 tbsp rice vinegar
- 1 tsp honey
- 1 tsp grated ginger
- 1/4 cup warm water
- 2 tbsp chopped cilantro (optional)
- Lime wedges for serving

Instructions:

1. In a large skillet or wok, heat the sesame oil over medium•high heat. Add the tofu cubes and cook, turning occasionally, until lightly browned on all sides, about 5•7 minutes. Transfer the tofu to a plate.

2. In the same skillet, add the broccoli, carrots, bell pepper, and garlic. Sauté for 5•7 minutes, until the vegetables are tender•crisp.

3. In a small bowl, whisk together the peanut butter, soy sauce, rice vinegar, honey, and ginger. Slowly whisk in the warm water until the sauce is smooth and creamy.

4. Add the cooked tofu back to the skillet with the vegetables. Pour the peanut sauce over the top and toss gently to coat everything evenly.

5. Serve the tofu and vegetables over steamed rice or noodles. Garnish with chopped cilantro and serve with lime wedges.

Enjoy this flavorful and nutritious tofu dish! The peanut sauce adds a delicious nutty and slightly sweet flavor that complements the vegetables and tofu perfectly.

113. Baked chicken with pesto

Ingredients:

- 4 boneless, skinless chicken breasts
- 1/2 cup prepared basil pesto
- 1/4 cup grated Parmesan cheese
- Salt and pepper to taste

Instructions:

1. Preheat your oven to 400°F (200°C). Lightly grease a baking dish or line a baking sheet with parchment paper.

2. Pat the chicken breasts dry with paper towels and season them with salt and pepper on both sides.

3. Spread about 2 tablespoons of pesto evenly over the top of each chicken breast, making sure to cover the entire surface.

4. Sprinkle the grated Parmesan cheese over the pesto•coated chicken.

5. Bake the chicken for 25•30 minutes, or until the internal temperature reaches 165°F (75°C) and the chicken is cooked through.

6. Remove the baked chicken from the oven and let it rest for 5 minutes before serving.

Serve the baked chicken with pesto warm, alongside your favorite sides like roasted vegetables, salad, or pasta.

Tips:
- Use a high•quality, store•bought pesto or make your own homemade pesto for the best flavor.
- Adjust the baking time based on the thickness of your chicken breasts.
- You can also broil the chicken for the last 2•3 minutes to get a nice golden•brown crust on top.
- For extra flavor, you can add a sprinkle of dried herbs, such as oregano or thyme, to the pesto before baking.

This baked chicken with pesto is a simple, yet delicious and healthy dinner option. The pesto and Parmesan cheese create a flavorful crust on the chicken, making it a crowd•pleasing meal.

114. Protein•infused oatmeal

Ingredients:

- 1 cup old•fashioned oats
- 1 scoop protein powder (vanilla or unflavored)
- 1 cup milk of your choice (dairy, almond, soy, etc.)
- 1/2 cup water
- 1 tbsp nut butter (peanut, almond, etc.)
- 1 tsp honey or maple syrup (optional)
- Pinch of cinnamon (optional)
- Toppings of your choice (berries, nuts, seeds, etc.)

Instructions:

1. In a medium saucepan, combine the oats, protein powder, milk, and water. Stir to combine.

2. Bring the mixture to a boil over medium heat, then reduce heat to low and let simmer for 5•7 minutes, stirring occasionally, until the oats are cooked through and have reached your desired consistency.

3. Remove from heat and stir in the nut butter until well combined.

4. Drizzle with honey or maple syrup if desired, and sprinkle with cinnamon.

5. Transfer to a bowl and top with your favorite toppings like fresh berries, nuts, seeds, etc.

The protein powder adds an extra boost of protein to keep you feeling full and satisfied. You can use any type of protein powder you prefer • whey, plant•based, etc. Adjust the amount of liquid to reach your desired oatmeal texture. Enjoy!

115. Turkey and avocado wrap

Ingredients:

- 4 whole wheat tortillas or wraps
- 8 oz sliced turkey breast
- 1 avocado, sliced
- 1 cup baby spinach or arugula
- 1/4 cup shredded cheddar or pepper jack cheese
- 2 tbsp hummus or Greek yogurt
- 1 tbsp olive oil
- Salt and pepper to taste

Instructions:

1. Lay the tortillas or wraps out on a clean surface.

2. Divide the turkey slices evenly among the 4 wraps, placing them in the center.

3. Top the turkey with sliced avocado, spinach/arugula, and shredded cheese.

4. Spread 1/2 tbsp of hummus or Greek yogurt onto each wrap.

5. Drizzle 1/4 tbsp of olive oil over the fillings on each wrap.

6. Season with salt and pepper to taste.

7. Fold the bottom of the wrap up over the fillings, then fold in the sides and continue rolling tightly into a burrito shape.

8. Slice the wraps in half diagonally and serve.

Tips:
- Use your favorite type of sliced turkey, such as smoked, roasted, or honey•roasted.
- Swap the hummus for mashed avocado or a creamy dressing if desired.
- Add other veggies like tomatoes, onions, or bell peppers.
- For extra protein, add a hard•boiled egg or cooked bacon.
- Wrap the finished wraps in parchment paper or foil to make them portable.

This turkey and avocado wrap is a delicious and nutritious lunch or snack. The combination of lean protein, healthy fats, and fresh veggies makes it a satisfying and well•balanced meal.

116. Eggplant lasagna with ground turkey

Ingredients:

- 2 medium eggplants, sliced lengthwise into 1/4•inch thick slices
- 1 lb ground turkey
- 1 onion, diced
- 3 cloves garlic, minced
- 1 (28 oz) can crushed tomatoes
- 1 tsp dried oregano
- 1 tsp dried basil
- Salt and pepper to taste
- 1 1/2 cups ricotta cheese
- 1 egg
- 1 cup shredded mozzarella cheese
- 1/2 cup grated Parmesan cheese

Instructions:

1. Preheat oven to 375°F. Lightly grease a 9x13 baking dish.

2. In a large skillet over medium heat, cook the ground turkey, onion, and garlic until the turkey is browned and cooked through, 5•7 minutes. Drain any excess fat.

3. Add the crushed tomatoes, oregano, basil, salt and pepper. Simmer for 10 minutes.

4. In a small bowl, mix together the ricotta cheese and egg until well combined.

5. Layer half the eggplant slices in the bottom of the prepared baking dish. Top with half the ricotta mixture, half the turkey tomato sauce, and 1/2 cup of the mozzarella cheese.

6. Repeat the layers one more time, ending with the remaining mozzarella and Parmesan cheeses.

7. Bake for 35•40 minutes, until the cheese is melted and bubbly. Let stand 10 minutes before serving.

Enjoy this healthy, veggie•packed lasagna! The eggplant slices make a great low•carb noodle substitute.

117. Baked chicken wings with a side of veggies

Ingredients:

Chicken Wings:
• 2 lbs chicken wings, drumettes and flats separated
• 2 tbsp olive oil
• 1 tsp garlic powder
• 1 tsp paprika
• 1/2 tsp salt
• 1/4 tsp black pepper

Veggie Side:
• 2 cups broccoli florets
• 1 cup baby carrots
• 1 red bell pepper, sliced
• 1 tbsp olive oil
• 1 tsp dried oregano
• Salt and pepper to taste

Instructions:

1. Preheat your oven to 400°F (200°C). Line a large baking sheet with parchment paper.

2. In a large bowl, toss the chicken wings with the olive oil, garlic powder, paprika, salt, and pepper until evenly coated.

3. Arrange the chicken wings in a single layer on the prepared baking sheet.

4. Bake the wings for 40•45 minutes, flipping halfway, until golden brown and cooked through.

5. While the wings are baking, prepare the veggie side. In a separate bowl, toss the broccoli, carrots, and bell pepper with the olive oil, oregano, salt, and pepper.

6. Spread the seasoned veggies on a separate baking sheet.

7. During the last 15 minutes of the chicken wings' baking time, add the veggie tray to the oven and bake both trays until the veggies are tender•crisp.

8. Remove the chicken wings and veggies from the oven. Serve the baked chicken wings hot, with the roasted veggies on the side.

This baked chicken wings and roasted veggie combo makes for a delicious and nutritious meal. The crispy wings paired with the tender, flavorful veggies is a winning combination.

118. Shrimp scampi with zucchini noodles

Ingredients:

- 1 lb large shrimp, peeled and deveined
- 3 tbsp unsalted butter
- 3 cloves garlic, minced
- 1/4 cup dry white wine
- 2 tbsp freshly squeezed lemon juice
- 1/4 cup chopped fresh parsley
- Salt and pepper to taste
- 3 medium zucchini, spiralized or julienned into noodles

Instructions:

1. In a large skillet, melt the butter over medium heat. Add the minced garlic and cook for 1 minute, until fragrant.

2. Add the shrimp to the skillet and cook for 2•3 minutes per side, until they start to turn pink and curl up. Transfer the shrimp to a plate and set aside.

3. Add the white wine and lemon juice to the skillet, scraping up any browned bits from the bottom of the pan. Let the sauce simmer for 2•3 minutes to reduce slightly.

4. Return the cooked shrimp to the skillet and toss to coat with the sauce. Stir in the chopped parsley and season with salt and pepper to taste.

5. Add the zucchini noodles to the skillet and toss gently to combine with the shrimp and sauce. Cook for 2•3 minutes, just until the zucchini noodles are tender but still have a bite.

6. Serve the shrimp scampi with zucchini noodles immediately, garnished with extra parsley if desired.

Tips:
- Use a spiralizer or julienne peeler to create the zucchini noodles.
- For a creamier sauce, stir in 2•3 tablespoons of heavy cream or half•and•half at the end.
- Substitute the white wine with chicken or vegetable broth if preferred.
- Add a pinch of red pepper flakes for a little heat.
- Serve with a side salad or crusty bread for a complete meal.

This shrimp scampi with zucchini noodles is a delicious and low•carb alternative to traditional pasta. The bright, garlicky sauce complements the tender shrimp and zucchini noodles perfectly.

119. Beef taco lettuce wraps

Ingredients:

- 1 lb ground beef
- 1 packet taco seasoning
- 1/2 cup water
- 12•16 large lettuce leaves (such as romaine or bibb)
- Toppings: diced tomatoes, shredded cheese, diced avocado, sour cream, salsa, etc.

Instructions:

1. In a large skillet over medium•high heat, cook the ground beef until browned and crumbled, about 5•7 minutes. Drain any excess fat.

2. Add the taco seasoning and water to the skillet with the ground beef. Stir to combine and let the mixture simmer for 5•7 minutes, or until the sauce has thickened.

3. Remove the skillet from heat and let the beef mixture cool slightly.

4. Lay out the lettuce leaves on a flat surface. Spoon the seasoned ground beef into the center of each lettuce leaf.

5. Top the beef with your desired toppings, such as diced tomatoes, shredded cheese, diced avocado, sour cream, and salsa.

6. Fold the lettuce leaves around the fillings and serve immediately.

These beef taco lettuce wraps are a delicious and low•carb alternative to traditional taco shells or tortillas. The crisp lettuce leaves provide a refreshing and crunchy base for the flavorful taco filling.

You can customize the toppings to your liking, adding more vegetables, different types of cheese, or even black beans or corn.

These lettuce wrap tacos are a great option for a healthy and satisfying meal. Serve them with a side of roasted vegetables or a fresh salad for a complete and balanced dinner.

Enjoy these easy and delicious beef taco lettuce wraps!

120. Chicken breast with tomato and basil

Ingredients:

- 4 boneless, skinless chicken breasts
- 2 tbsp olive oil
- 2 cloves garlic, minced
- 1 (14.5 oz) can diced tomatoes
- 1/4 cup fresh basil leaves, chopped
- 1/4 tsp red pepper flakes (optional)
- Salt and pepper to taste

Instructions:

1. Season the chicken breasts with salt and pepper on both sides.

2. In a large skillet, heat the olive oil over medium•high heat. Add the chicken breasts and cook for 5•7 minutes per side, or until they are golden brown and cooked through. Transfer the chicken to a plate and set aside.

3. In the same skillet, add the minced garlic and sauté for 1 minute, until fragrant.

4. Add the diced tomatoes (with their juices) to the skillet. Bring the mixture to a simmer and cook for 3•5 minutes, stirring occasionally, until the sauce has thickened slightly.

5. Stir in the chopped fresh basil and red pepper flakes (if using). Season with additional salt and pepper to taste.

6. Return the cooked chicken breasts to the skillet, nestling them into the tomato•basil sauce.

7. Reduce the heat to low and let the chicken simmer in the sauce for 5•10 minutes, or until the chicken is heated through and the flavors have melded.

8. Serve the chicken breasts immediately, spooning the tomato•basil sauce over the top.

This chicken breast with tomato and basil is a simple, yet flavorful dish. The juicy chicken is complemented by the fresh, vibrant tomato•basil sauce. The red pepper flakes add a subtle heat, but you can omit them if you prefer a milder dish.

Serve this chicken with a side of roasted vegetables, a fresh salad, or a serving of whole grain rice or pasta for a complete and balanced meal. Enjoy!